Moving from Your Associate to Your Baccalaureate Nursing Degree

First Edition

Nancy H. Duphily, DNP

Fitchburg State University

D1294406

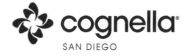

cognella®

SAN DIEGO

Bassim Hamadeh, CEO and Publisher
John Remington, Executive Editor
Gem Rabanera, Senior Project Editor
Abbey Hastings, Production Editor
Emely Villavicencio, Senior Graphic Designer
Kylie Bartolome, Licensing Associate
Natalie Piccotti, Director of Marketing
Kassie Graves, Senior Vice President, Editorial
Jamie Giganti, Director of Academic Publishing

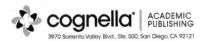

3970 Sorrento Valley Blvd., Ste. 500, San Diego, CA 92121

CONTENTS

Acknowledgments   xi
Introduction   xv

Chapter 1.   Succeed in Your Nursing Education Program   **1**

Chapter Introduction   1

Key Terms : Making Connections   1

Learning Objectives/Outcomes   2

A Nurse's Perspective   2

In Pursuit of a Bachelor of Science in Nursing (BSN):
Current Status of Nursing in the United States   3

Choosing the RN to BSN Pathway   4

Professional Organizations   5

Professional Standards   6

Foundational Documents of Professional Nursing   7

From Novice to Expert: Benner's Stages of Clinical Competence   10

A Nurse's Perspective   10

A Word About Writing Skills   11

Chapter Summary   12

Food for Thought: Critical Thinking Questions   13

Scenarios: Applying What You Have Learned   13

Nursing Journal: Reflect on Your Practice While
Honing Your Writing Skills   14

Chapter 1 References   14

Other Resources   16

Chapter 2.   Disseminate Knowledge and Caring   **17**

Chapter Introduction   17

Key Terms : Making Connections   17

Learning Objectives/Outcomes   18

A Nurse's Perspective   18

Disseminate Knowledge   18

Research Translation Barriers   19

Disseminating Research Knowledge   19

Disseminating Caring   20

Clinical Significance of the Code of Ethics   21

Ethical Dilemmas   21

Ethics and Civility in Nursing   22

Chapter Summary   26

Food for Thought: Critical Thinking Questions   27

Scenario: Applying What You Have Learned   27

Nursing Journal: Reflect on Your Practice While
Honing Your Writing Skills   28

Chapter 2 References   28

Chapter 3.   Provide Patient-Centered Care   **32**

Chapter Introduction   32

Key Terms: Making Connections   32

Learning Objectives/Outcomes   33

A Nurse's Perspective   33

The Science of Providing Patient-Centered
Care: The Picker Institute   34

Overview of Picker's Eight Principles of Patient-Centered Care   35

Nursing Education Reform   36

Nursing Theories Related to Patient-Centered Care   38

Person-Centered Care: Theory in Practice   42

Patient-Centered Care: Implications for Nursing Practice   43

Fostering Patient Participation in Decision Making   44

Transparency in Communication   45

Social Determinants of Health   45

Healthy People 2020   47

Providing Culturally Sensitive Care   47

Chapter Summary   48

Food for Thought: Critical Thinking Questions   48

Scenario: Culturally Sensitive Care   49

Nursing Journal: Reflect on Your Practice While
Honing Your Writing Skills   49

Chapter 3 References   50

Additional Resources   52

Chapter 4.   Work in Interprofessional Teams   53

Chapter Introduction   53

Key Terms: Making Connections   53

Learning Objectives/Outcomes   54

A Nurse's Perspective   54

The IOM Report and Interprofessional Collaboration   55

Interprofessional Practice and Education   55

The Interprofessional Team   57

Interprofessional Health-Care Challenges   57

Promoting the Interprofessional Team in Health Care   57

Nurse Leadership, Collaboration, and Healthy Work Environments   58

Interprofessional Care Teams: King's Theory of Goal Attainment   59

Shared Governance   60

Effective Communication Tools in Providing Safe
Patient Care: The Handoff Report   62

The SBAR (Situation, Background, Assessment,
Recommendation) Handoff   63

I-PASS: Illness Severity/Patient Summary/Action List/
Situation Awareness and Contingency Plans   64

Bedside Shift Report (BSR)   65

Chapter Summary   67

Food for Thought: Critical Thinking Questions   67

Scenario: Applying What You Have Learned   67

Nursing Journal: Reflect on Your Practice While
Honing Your Writing Skills   68

Chapter 4 References   69

Chapter 5.   Employ Evidence-Based Practice   **71**

Chapter Introduction   71

Key Terms: Making Connections   71

Learning Objectives/Outcomes   72

A Nurse's Perspective   72

EBP in Nursing   73

EBP in Nursing: Origins   74

Levels of EBP: Rating Systems   75

Evidence Hierarchy Ratings   76

Implementing the Evidence   76

How Does EBP Benefit Nurses and Patients?   77

Educating Nursing Students About EBP   77

The PICOT Model (Population, Intervention, Comparison, Outcome, and Time)   78

Examples of PICOT Questions   79

Reading and Critiquing a Research Article   79

Linking Evidence to Practice: The Clinical Practice Guideline Project   81

The Literature Search   83

Critically Appraising the Evidence   83

Comparing Recommendations to Actual Practice: The Iowa Model   84

Evaluation   84

Implications and Recommendations   86

Implications of EBP for the Nursing Profession   87

Chapter Summary   87

Food for Thought: Critical Thinking Questions   87

Scenario: Applying What you Have Learned   88

Nursing Journal: Reflect on Your Practice While Honing Your Writing Skills   88

Chapter 5 References   89

Chapter 6.   Apply Quality Improvement (QI)   **91**

Chapter Introduction   91

Key Terms: Making Connections   91

Learning Objectives/Outcomes   92

A Nurse's Perspective   92

Lewin's Change Theory   93

Unfreezing, Change, and Refreezing   93

The Lean Model   94

QI   95

The Four Steps of QI   96

Model for Improvement: PDSA   97

Example of a Test of Change (PDSA Cycle)   98

Lactation Management Team, Postpartum Breastfeeding Mother   98

QSEN   100

A Just Culture of Safety   101

Chapter Summary   102

Food for Thought: Critical Thinking   102

Scenario: Applying What You Have Learned   103

Nursing Journal: Reflect on Your Practice While
Honing Your Writing Skills   103

Chapter 6 References   104

Other References   105

Chapter 7.   Utilize Informatics   106

Chapter Introduction   106

Key Terms: Making Connections   106

Learning Objectives/Outcomes   107

A Nurse's Perspective   107

Nursing Informatics   107

Kotter's Change Management Theory   109

The Role of Informatics Technology in Transforming Health Care   110

The Nurse Informatics Specialist   111

Telehealth and Telenursing   114

Nursing and HIPAA   116

Chapter Summary   117

Food for Thought: Critical Thinking Questions   118

Scenario: Applying What You Have Learned   118

Nursing Journal: Reflect on Your Practice While
Honing Your Writing Skills   119

Chapter 7 References   119

ACCESSING WEB-BASED RESOURCES

This book has QR codes available to complement your reading.

The author has selected additional web-based content for further engagement using QR codes, which are intended for those who have purchased print copies of the book. Those who have purchased a digital copy may simply click on the corresponding hyperlinks. Please check with your professor to confirm whether your class will access this content independently or collectively.

Cognella maintains no responsibility for the content nor availability of third-party links. However, Cognella makes every effort to keep texts current. Broken links may be reported to studentreviews@cognella.com. Please include the book's title, author, and 7-digit SKU reference number (found below the barcode on the back cover of the book) in the body of your message.

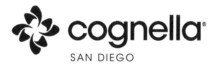

Acknowledgments

A THANK YOU TO OUR NURSES

To comfort and advocate ... that is what nurses do in any role they take on. And for me, that role is a privilege.

—Kathleen Trieb, RN, University of Vermont Medical Center

I would be remiss if I did not point out that this book was written during the COVID-19 pandemic. The series of events that transpired following the March 2020 outbreak produced many new and conflicting emotions, from anxiety, disbelief, and terror, to sadness, hope, and optimism. In "remote" conversations with friends, relatives, colleagues, and students, it was apparent that many of us shared similar conflicting emotions during this crisis—emotions that appeared to change on a daily basis. We found what strategies helped weather the storm, and what did not.

For me, creating this work became a source of inspiration and pride in the nursing profession. Ironically, as the world fell apart around us, this moment in time instilled a greater sense of appreciation of and gratitude for the profession I have known for over 40 years. Composing each chapter while teaching students in the online RN to BS *Transitions* course during self-imposed isolation was an invaluable experience. Communicating the stories of nurses, both past and present, celebrating their daily workplace challenges and victories, and acknowledging the contributions being brought to the academic table are the primary messages I hope to convey to readers.

The following are just two examples of the many heroic acts of our RN to BS nursing students working on the front lines of the COVID-19 pandemic:

> I work in a hospital that is currently preparing for a COVID-19 surge. I am one of the COVID nurses, meaning I care for COVID rule outs as well as COVID positive patients. The patient load is currently low and slow. I am actually grateful for this, as each shift I work the policies and procedures change (specifically relating to PPE), as I am sure many nurses can relate to especially in these times. There are so many incidents that I could speak of ... too many. The one that is forefront and current in my mind is the decision I

had to make on a personal level. I have a son that lives with me, and to keep him safe I had to have him stay with his father and isolate from him. My gut was twisted in knots, all pertaining to the stress level I felt having to go home and possibly expose my son. This was creating so much negativity in my nursing practice. For me, the critical incident was the decision that was not only safest for my son but in the best interests of my patients. This decision was critical for my ability to perform at my highest level and focus on the critical level of care needed. Nursing theorist Hildegard Peplau maintains that the kind of person the nurse becomes makes a substantial difference in what each patient will learn while receiving nursing care. Peplau's theory explains roles and methods in nursing as an interpersonal process. Specifically meaningful to me is the Identification phase, which relates to exploring the needs of the patient and the importance of the nurse assisting patients with their feelings while sustaining a positive environment. The COVID-19 pandemic is one that has created such fear, not only with our patients but also with healthcare workers. It is imperative to maintain a positive environment at all times for the health and wellness for all involved. Understanding that being away from my son is not a positive it has created an environment to enable me to focus on my patients' environment and needs. Peplau's framework for therapeutic behavior of nurses aided in identifying ways to decrease anxiety and stress in patients. I was unaware of the impact making the decision I did was going to have on my nursing practice but it has. I am focused. I am determined. I am positive in knowing we will get through this.

I never thought that I'd be on the front lines of a pandemic in my first year as a nurse. This pandemic has rattled many of us in ways we have never experienced before. It's brought a lot of fear and uncertainty. I work in acute care on a Respiratory unit and treat many COVID-19 patients. Despite some of the challenges that I've faced (i.e., lack of PPE), I am heartened by the amazing support of my colleagues. Whenever I'm in a patient's room, with full protective equipment on, I can always count on my colleagues to gather the supplies I need. This pandemic has really shown me the importance of teamwork. It has allowed me to overcome many obstacles. It has also reminded me of the reason I decided to pursue a career in the medical field. My will to help people and care for them drives me through this crisis. This pandemic has made me realize how important caring is in the nursing profession, and it has led me to the works of Jean Watson. Jean Watson is an American nurse theorist who is known for her "Philosophy and Theory of Transpersonal

Caring." She believes that caring is essential to the nursing practice. Caring is the essence of nursing and with the various demands of the nursing field, it can be difficult to lose sight of it.

Although life as we know it may have changed, the fundamental nature of nurses has not waivered. Nurses will always prevail in providing the human connection patients need to help them heal. Our thoughts turn to those serving on the front lines of the COVID-19 pandemic. Unable to shelter-in-place with their own families or to stay 6 feet away from sick patients, their actions reveal the substantial role nurses and other health-care providers play in society. We rely on their courage and sacrifices when facing unexpected turmoil each shift, only to return the next day to repeat the same actions.

Nurses demonstrate the remarkable ability to support others during their own individual periods of vulnerability. To risk peril in their work so that others may stay safe at home demands an uncommon degree of selflessness and bravery. During this unparalleled time of fear and uncertainty, we thank our noble heroes.

Nancy Duphily
April 2020

Introduction

THE ASSOCIATE DEGREE NURSE PURSUING A BACCALAUREATE DEGREE

In 2017, the American Association of Colleges of Nursing (AACN, 2017) circulated a draft position calling for the bachelor of science in nursing (BSN) to become the minimum preparation for professional nursing practice. As more than half of nursing enrollment toward becoming a registered nurse (RN) originates from the associate degree nursing (ADN) program (NCSBNa; NCSBN 2018c; NCSBNd;), the National League for Nursing, American Association of Community Colleges, and the Association of Community College Trustees raised their opposition to the AACN position (2018). The AACN (2019a) then reiterated its commitment toward the educational progression of ADNs to the BSN (RN-BSN) as a replacement for their original stance of BSN-only nursing (Sabio & Petges, 2020).

The primary reasons for the emphasis on higher levels of education for the nursing workforce relate to the growing complexity of patient care as a result of medical and technological advances and the expanding scopes of practice and role of nurses in managing patients and the health-care system (Institute of Medicine [IOM], 2011; Sabio & Petges, 2020).

Different avenues have been proposed and opened to help achieve higher educational attainment for nurses. Because more than half of nurses graduate from the ADN program, RN-BSN education has been the most popular, resulting in the growth in RN-BSN completion rates (Buerhaus et al., 2016; National League for Nursing, 2016; Shen et al., 2015). Despite this progress, the goal of 80% BSN by 2020 (Altman et al., 2016) is unlikely to be met. Although ADNs are progressing to the BSN level at an all-time high, there remains a large number of incumbent RNs without a BSN (Spetz, 2018).

In their qualitative study, Sabio and Petges (2020) interviewed ADN students to examine and understand their perceived barriers to BSN education. Factors such as time management and balancing the demands of family, work, and school were recurrent themes. In addition, students identified financial aid issues, lack of additional assistance, class schedules, and too much content and "busy work" in their nursing curriculum (Sabio & Petges, 2020).

The ADN response to the question as to what would lower barriers to achieving a baccalaureate degree in nursing revealed the theme of *making classes more accessible and flexible* (Sabio & Petges, 2020). The online platform appealed to this population, as it provided them with the opportunity to attend to their responsibilities at home and work while pursuing their BSN degrees at a pace more agreeable to their lifestyles:

> Online classes give more choices …. That one less day that I need to drive to school and sit in class for 3 hours and figure out what my kids are going to do and what I'm doing for dinner, I can nap, and I can work night shift. I can do my homework and listen to my lectures at 3 in the morning, because I'm awake—having that kind of flexibility. I think online is 100% beneficial for certain demographics of people.

According to the authors (Sabio & Petges, 2020), current literature has revealed scarce research related to the challenges that ADN students face in advancing their nursing education. Feedback from their ADN focus group interviews was significant on many levels. The process highlighted major themes associated with barriers to achieving the BSN, revealed a possible connection between barriers and the nontraditional characteristics of the ADN, and provided insight into removing these obstacles. Understanding these variables could prove particularly helpful in creating strategies to streamline a realistic quality educational pathway for the ADN seeking a baccalaureate degree in nursing.

THE FORMAT OF THIS BOOK

Scaffolding

This textbook introduces the reader to the instructional technology strategy of *scaffolding* knowledge. *Transitions* incorporates the interactive, progressive building of knowledge. Integrated throughout this process is the opportunity to practice and refine skills in the areas of self-reflection, critical thinking, writing mechanics, American Psychological Association format, leadership, and communication.

In these pages, readers will choose a concept of interest, develop a PICOT question, search the literature, and critique a selected article to determine if it is, indeed, "scholarly." In addition, readers will recall a "critical incident" and examine which, if any, nursing theorists/theories align with their current practice. Quotes from nursing leaders, nursing theorists, and members of the interdisciplinary health-care team, as well as stories from practicing nurses, exemplify and support current evidence in the profession. Chapter exercises provide readers the time and opportunity to reflect on their professional practice.

Scaffolding is an important concept that allows for a continuous structured learning experience. It is intended that students/readers will appreciate the model as an introduction for nurses exposed for the first time to the online educational experience. Each chapter builds on the other by reinforcing ideas, with the opportunity to reflect on the chapter's main ideas by way of critical thinking and writing exercises. These tools help students to delve deeper into the initial idea presented in each chapter. Scaffolding knowledge reinforces ideas through the various connections presented. The process is intended to keep the main idea in focus but allow for constant reflection, refinement of ideas, and personal and professional growth.

AN EXPLANATION OF WHAT TO EXPECT IN EACH SECTION OF THE TEXT

Literature Search

Most nurses today will be required to complete a literature review at some point, either as part of a course of study, as a key step in the research process, or as part of clinical practice development or policy. For student nurses and novice researchers, it is often seen as a difficult undertaking. It demands a complex range of skills, such as learning how to define topics for exploration, acquiring skills for literature searching and retrieval, developing the ability to analyze and synthesize data, and becoming adept at writing and reporting, often within a limited timescale.

The Critical Incident

A critical incident is one in which you believe the intervention made a difference in a patient outcome, either directly or indirectly. It may include the following: an incident that went unusually well, an incident in which there was a breakdown (things did not go as planned), an incident that captured the epitome of what nursing is all about, or an incident that was particularly demanding. Give a detailed description of what happened. Why was this incident "critical"? What were the concerns at the time? What was particularly demanding or satisfying? A critical incident is one that causes us to pause and contemplate the events that have occurred to try to give them some meaning. Using a critical incident as a way of reflecting involves the identification of behavior thought to have been particularly helpful or unhelpful in a given situation. Almost everyone at some time considers how things could have been avoided, overcome, or improved. Good research projects often start with the identification of a problem, and those projects, which solve or eliminate clinical problems, are the most worthwhile. The answers to nursing research questions help nurses provide more effective nursing care and document the unique role nursing plays in the health-care system.

SCENARIOS: APPLYING WHAT YOU HAVE LEARNED

Nursing scenarios convey everyday realistic, complex situations. They often involve a dilemma, conflict, or problem that individuals involved must resolve. Scenarios bridge the gap between theory and practice, classroom and workplace. In addition, they provide an opportunity to practice skills in problem identification, discuss differing viewpoints, and evaluate alternative courses of action. In this way, the scenario approach helps students integrate, apply and refine clinical reasoning, critical thinking, and problem-solving skills. Scenarios are intended to reinforce and supplement (scaffold) your learning.

FOOD FOR THOUGHT: CRITICAL THINKING QUESTIONS

The "*Food for Thought*" sections at the end of each chapter summarize the main concepts of the particular lesson. When you relate a story of a memorable experience, you summarize. When you give a brief oral report on a current magazine article, you summarize. Occasionally, an instructor may ask you to summarize in writing something you have read. This section is intended to help you recognize the important points made in the assigned readings. Summarizing is about extracting the main ideas and major support while omitting the rest. Lesson recaps, posed as questions, play a crucial role in helping you develop and synthesize the highlights of the assigned readings, leading to a deeper understanding of what the author is saying.

CRITIQUING A JOURNAL ARTICLE

For any type of journal article, your critique/comparison should include some basic information:

- Author/s
- Title of article
- Title of journal (include volume numbers/dates/months/page numbers)
- Statement of the problem or issues
- Purpose, methods, hypothesis, major conclusions

Read the article once to get an overview. Then read it again, critically, answering the following questions:

- Is the article title appropriate and clear?
- Is the purpose of the article made clear in the introduction?
- Is the discussion relevant?
- Has the author cited pertinent literature?
- Should some sections of the manuscript be expanded/condensed/omitted?
- Are the author's statements clear?
- Has the author been objective in the discussion of the topic?

WHAT IS A PICOT?

Writing a well-developed question makes the rest of the process of finding and evaluating evidence easier. When you determine the outcome, it helps you hone the process of searching for evidence. Evidence is not just what you want the outcome to be; it is evaluating the evidence, supporting or refuting what influences the outcome.

- **P:** Population/disease
- **I:** Intervention or variable of interest
- **C:** Comparison
- **O:** Outcome
- **T:** Time

This textbook sets the groundwork for the ADN returning to the academic arena in pursuit of a baccalaureate degree. Individual chapters align with IOM competencies and emphasize leadership and management, critical thinking, evidence-based research, communication, and self-reflective skills, all supported by literature and practice examples. As future change agents, the reader is able to reflect on current issues and trends that are influencing nursing education and practice. In addition, the text lays the foundation upon which the reader can examine and build on those skills that were introduced in their respective entry-level nursing programs. It is anticipated that the information in this book will enable the reader to comprehend those processes inherent in the successful transition to the role of the baccalaureate-prepared nurse.

REFERENCES

Altman, S., Butler, A., & Shern, L. (2016). *Assessing progress on the Institute of Medicine report: The future of nursing.* The National Academies Press.

American Association of Colleges of Nursing (AACN). (2017). *The baccalaureate degree as entry-level preparation for professional nursing practice.* http://www.aacnnursing.org/News-Information/News/View/ArticleId/20690/Academic-Progression-Task-Force-Seeks-Feedback-on-Position-Statement

American Association of Colleges of Nursing (AACN). (2019a). *Academic progression in nursing: Moving together toward a highly educated nursing workforce.* https://www.aacnnursing.org/News-Information/Position-Statements-White-Papers/Academic-Progression-in-Nursing

American Association of Colleges of Nursing (AACN). (2019b). *American Association of Colleges of Nursing Fact sheet: Nursing shortage.* https://www.aacnnursing.org/Portals/42/News/Factsheets/Nursing-Shortage-Factsheet.pdf

Buerhaus, P., Auerbach, D. & Stager, D. (2016). Data watch. Recent changes in the number of nurses graduating from undergraduate and graduate programs. *Nursing Economic$, 34* (1),46–48.

Institute of Medicine (IOM). (2011). *The future of nursing: Focus on education.* http://www.iom.edu/Reports/2010/The-Future-of-Nursing-Leading-Change-Advancing-Health/Report-Brief-Education.aspx?page=1

National Council of State Boards of Nursing. (2018a). Enhanced nurse licensure compact (eNLC) implemented Jan. 19, 2018. Retrieved from https://ncsbn.org/11945.htm

National Council of State Boards of Nursing. (2018c). Nurse licensure compact (NLC). Retrieved from https://www.ncsbn.org/nurse-licensurecompact.htm

National Council of State Boards of Nursing. (2018d). The national nursing database: A profile of nursing licensure in the US. Retrieved from https://www.ncsbn.org/national-nursing-database.htm

National League for Nursing. (2016). *Percentage of students enrolled by program type, 2015–2016.* http://www.nln.org/docs/default-source/newsroom/nursing-education-statistics/percentage-of-qualified-applications-turned-away-by-program-type-2016-(pdf).pdf?sfvrsn=0

National League for Nursing. (2018). National league for nursing responds to AACN draft vision statement for future of nursing education. Retrieved from http://www.nln.org/newsroom/news-releases/news-release/2018/06/11/national-league-fornursing-responds-to-aacn-draft-vision-statement-for-future-of-nursing-education

Sabio, C., & Petges, N. (2020). Understanding the barriers to BSN education among ADN students: A qualitative study. *Teaching and Learning in Nursing, 15*(1), 45–52. https://doi.org/10.1016/j.teln.2019.08.007

Shen, Q., PeltzerJ., Teel, C., & Pierce, J. (2015). The initiative to move toward a more highly educated nursing workforce: Findings from the Kansas registered nurse workforce survey. *Journal of Professional Nursing, 31* (6), 452.

Spetz, J. (2018). Projections of progress toward the 80% bachelor of science in nursing: Recommendation and strategies to accelerate change. *Nursing Outlook, 66* (4), 394–400.

CHAPTER 1

Succeed in Your Nursing Education Program

CHAPTER INTRODUCTION

The purpose of this chapter is to welcome and introduce the nurse returning to academia for a baccalaureate degree to the opportunities and responsibilities advanced education presents. A brief overview of the current status of health care in the United States, Code of Ethics, Scope and Standards of Practice, and Social Policy Statements are presented for the student's review of and reflection on their relevance and value in professional practice. The inclusion of Benner's *Novice to Expert Stages of Clinical Competence* compels students to identify personal and professional goals as they develop their knowledge and skills in their goal of becoming "experts." Concluding the chapter, readers are encouraged to practice and refine their writing skills as a link to success in advanced professional practice, effective leadership and management, and effecting evidence-based changes in practice.

KEY TERMS: MAKING CONNECTIONS

- Benner's stages of clinical competence
  - Novice
  - Advanced beginner
  - Competent
  - Proficient
  - Expert
- Code of ethics

- Professional nursing organizations
- Professional practice standards
- Writing skills

LEARNING OBJECTIVES/OUTCOMES

In this chapter, students will accomplish the following

- Examine the roles of professional nursing organizations that affect nursing education
- Discuss the relevance of standards to the nursing profession
- Describe Benner's stages of clinical competence
- Explain the purpose of the documents from the American Nurses Association's (ANA) Foundations of Nursing:
  - Code of Ethics for Nurses
  - Nursing: Scope and Standards of Practice
  - Nursing's Social Policy Statement
- Recognize the value of possessing quality writing skills in effecting change.

> Let us never consider ourselves finished nurses …
> we must be learning all of our lives.
>
> *Florence Nightingale*

A NURSE'S PERSPECTIVE

Provision 2 of the Code of Ethics for Nurses with Interpretive Statements explains that the nurse's primary commitment is to the patient. We cannot forget about ourselves, however. Provision 5.2 reminds us that we have to take the same care for our own health and safety (ANA, 2015a). When the marathon bombing took place, I was working at my current job in the ED at Boston Children's. The best way to describe the day was controlled chaos. A co-worker turned to me and she said, "I am afraid." I told her I was too. In that moment, we both realized that while we were both going through the motions, not skipping a beat, we both shared this mutual feeling of fear. I think sometimes we think we might be the only ones experiencing fear or uncertainty but once you talk with your co-workers, you realize that we all share these feelings. I think it is extremely important that we are open and honest with our feelings as we support one another. (RN to BS student)

IN PURSUIT OF A BACHELOR OF SCIENCE IN NURSING (BSN): CURRENT STATUS OF NURSING IN THE UNITED STATES

Nurses play a significant role in the U.S. health professions, as evidenced by the World Health Statistics report, which stated that of the 29 million nurses, 3.9 million reside in the United States (Slattery et al., 2016). Experts predict that one million additional nurses will be needed by 2020 (Aiken et al., 2003). The U.S. Bureau of Labor Statistics has projected that 11 million additional nurses are needed to avoid a major shortage. Employment opportunities for nurses are projected to grow at a faster rate (15%) than all other occupations from 2016 through 2026 (Haddad & Toney-Butler, 2019).

The causes related to the nursing shortage are many—from lack of nursing educators, high turnover rates, and staffing ratios, to inequitable distribution of the workforce—and of major concern (Halter et al. et al., 2017). Further confounding this problem is a rise in the number of aging Americans. *Baby boomers*, many with comorbidities, are in need of increased health care. The final population of baby boomers reaches retirement age in 2029, forecasting a 73% increase in Americans 65 years of age and older. This suggests an increased strain on both current health-care services and on an aging nursing workforce.

With approximately one million registered nurses (RNs) older than 50 years old, one third of the workforce will be at retirement age within the next decade. This number includes nursing faculty members, which presents the challenge of educating more nurses with fewer resources. A scarcity of nursing educators affects enrollment and ultimately restricts the numbers that a nursing school can graduate. A limited number of faculty members leads to fewer students, a decline in classes, an increased risk to program quality (Haddad & Toney-Butler, 2019), and, ultimately, fewer nurses in the pipeline to meet the impending shortage (Buerhaus et al., 2017).

According to AACN's 2018–2019 (2019a) report, *Enrollment and Graduations in Baccalaureate and Graduate Programs in Nursing*, U.S. nursing schools turned away 75,029 qualified applicants from baccalaureate and graduate nursing programs in 2018 because of an insufficient number of faculty, clinical sites and instructors, classroom space, and financial challenges. Nursing schools responding to a related AACN survey cited scarce faculty numbers for their inability to accept quality baccalaureate applicants into their programs. Efforts to reduce the faculty shortage include the creativity of four states (Hawaii, Georgia, Maryland, and Colorado), which created legislation to allocate $1.5 million per year to provide up to five $1,000 tax credits per clinical preceptor (AACN, 2019a).

Health care has changed significantly during the past decade, and with this change, opportunities for nurses have transformed. With more information, and more of this information to process, nurses need the education, experience, and expertise in technology to manage that information for safe quality patient care. A vital role for nurses is to ensure that the "right person is providing the right care for the patient at the right cost" (AACN, 2019a; 2019b).

CHOOSING THE RN TO BSN PATHWAY

The hospital is no longer the central focus of care. Nursing students are educated, and nurses practice in a multitude of diverse locations ranging from community centers and walk-in clinics to schools. Moreover, with the emphasis on health care related to health promotion and disease prevention, nurses are further challenged to assume a larger role in patient care.

For nurses returning to academia, the BSN degree provides a foundation on which to build a career through further study. Possessing a baccalaureate degree affords the recipient a clear pathway to pursue the goals of becoming an advanced practice RN. While the potential at this level is great, the responsibilities are even greater, supporting the need for progressive nursing education: "The increased complexity of health problems and increased management of health problems out of the hospitals require highly educated and well-prepared nurses at the baccalaureate and graduate level" (AACN, 2019b).

According to Romp et al. (2014), nurses return to academia with the goal of career advancement in leadership and education roles. Growing health-care challenges, shifting government regulations, and rapid technological innovations mean that nurses require additional education to keep up with job demands. Nurses who further their education are able to effect change directly by working in specialized high-need areas, such as informatics, critical care, and health-care policy.

For many, returning to academia requires careful, advanced preparation, which includes financial considerations and creative scheduling, to adapt to new school, work, and family obligations (Perfetto, 2015). Online nursing programs permit students to pursue their degrees part or full time while continuing to maintain the responsibilities of home, family, and work. Many programs provide online learners with financial incentives through discounted tuition or residency waivers (Osterman et al., 2009).

A qualitative systematic review was conducted by Anbari (2015), who sought to develop a model outlining the process of RNs returning to obtain a BSN. In this process, Anbari asked the following questions: (a) What antecedents

See key findings on the *Distance Education Enrollment Report* by clicking on this link:

https://onlinelearningconsortium.org/read/digital-learning-compass-distance-education-enrollment-report-2017/

Or you can use your cell phone to scan the QR code and access the article:

must exist prior to returning to school to earn a BSN degree? (b) What occurs while attending an RN to BSN program? (c) What do RNs identify as outcomes of earning a BSN degree? (d) Does a seamless transition for RNs to become BSNs exist?

Once they matriculated into such a program, RNs reported that this "transformative" journey was not without its challenges and remains an experience where support (family, professional, and institutional) is vital for academic success. They spoke positively of their educational experience, citing improvements in their daily nursing practice, along with a renewed interest in lifelong learning. Additional benefits included career mobility, enhanced critical thinking, improved collaboration with coworkers, and greater patient advocacy (Anbari, 2015).

Based on Anbari's (2015) findings, nurses contemplating a baccalaureate degree should first examine their motivation for returning to school. Other key recommendations include finding the right program at the right time, place, and price. Students, their workplaces, and their institutions of learning should continually evaluate their organizations' programs to address challenges faced by students, as well as to strategize about what barriers obstruct progress and which methods work best for student success.

The health-care industry is demanding more and more from nurses. The education of nurses must go beyond chemistry, anatomy, language, and mathematics to instill a more profound understanding of health promotion, disease prevention, and social determinants of health. Nurses must recognize that health problems often have socially contributing factors, such as poverty and the environment. Also, nurses must possess insight into those aspects of culture, values, and ethics that affect human behavior. As a challenging and exciting career, the nursing profession promises lifelong learning, continual individual growth, and exceptional experiences (Clifford et al., 2018).

PROFESSIONAL ORGANIZATIONS

Professional nursing organizations influence health-care policy, represent and protect the interests of nurses, provide continuing education opportunities, and advocate for the highest quality nursing care possible to the public. An example is the American Nursing Association (ANA), the largest of all the U.S. professional nursing organizations. The ANA represents the nursing profession and the interests of 3.4 million nurses. The ANA's stated mission is "nurses advancing our profession to improve the health of all" (Roux & Halstead, 2018).

Professional nursing organizations have the potential to positively transform nursing practice, nursing education, health policy, and health-care standards. Membership in organizations provides a means by which nurses can be involved in influencing health-care policy and effecting positive change. Participation in professional organizations fosters leadership development, enhances skills in collaboration, provides networking opportunities for each member, and leads to career advancement (Matthews, 2012).

Membership in Professional Organizations

Nurses account for the largest number of health-care workers in the United States (Haddad & Toney-Butler, 2019). Their voices have the potential to significantly affect health-care reform in the United States. However, the lack of nursing participation in national discussions restricts the accurate representation of the profession. This finding severely limits communication about the contributions made by the nursing profession to improve health care (Haddad & Toney-Butler, 2019).

Concerns about the lack of nursing representation on national health-care boards led to an initiative to place 10,000 nurses on national boards by the year 2020. Addressing the concern about the lack of nursing leadership in health care, the *Future of Nursing* report (Institute of Medicine [IOM], 2010) called for the nursing workforce to be prepared to lead change in health care. The IOM report specifically recommended that **professional nursing organizations** develop nurse leaders through mentoring and leadership development programs. In this way, nurses are able to develop skills by undertaking leadership roles within the organizations.

Catallo et al. (2014) conducted a systematic website review of professional nursing organizations to examine how they involved RNs in health policy activities. This study found that many nursing organizations are actively working to address nursing and health-care policy issues. However, the authors reported that continued work is needed to promote nursing engagement and to evaluate the effectiveness of those strategies employed by professional nursing organizations to support political activities.

PROFESSIONAL STANDARDS

Professional standards define competent levels of care in each component of the nursing process. The main purpose of **professional nursing standards** is to guide competent nursing practice. Standards provide an evaluation tool to ensure clinical proficiency and safety (Davis, 2014).

Professional nursing standards are also used to provide a framework for developing clinical competency checklists or proficiency evaluations for a specific clinical unit or employer. Professional standards assist nurses, nursing administrations, and health-care organizations to develop safe staffing practices, delegate tasks to licensed and unlicensed personnel, ensure adequate documentation, and even create policies for new technology, such as social media.

Violating a professional standard can expose the nurse and the affiliated health-care organization to liability and potential loss of licensure. Professional standards guarantee that nurses are accountable for their decisions and actions, as well as for maintaining competence during their careers. These standards encourage nurses to persistently enhance their knowledge base through experience, continuing education, and in following the latest guidelines. Nurses must continue to ensure that their clinical practice meets or exceeds established professional standards to maintain patients' trust and respect.

FOUNDATIONAL DOCUMENTS OF PROFESSIONAL NURSING

The ANA (2015a) has published three resources that inform nurses' thinking and decision making and guide their practice.

Nursing's Social Policy Statement. This statement (ANA, 2014c) defines nursing, conceptualizes nursing practice, and describes the social context of nursing.

Nursing: Scope and Standards of Practice (2010b). The document outlines the RN scope of practice; it represents standards and competencies that delineate the role of the professional nurse.

Code of Ethics for Nurses with Interpretive Statements (ANA, 2001a) is the ethical foundation for nurses across diverse roles and settings. *The Code of Ethics for Nurses with Interpretive Statements* is nursing's contract with patients to provide safe, quality care. It also fosters nurses' collegial support to meet ethical and professional obligations. The code is regularly reviewed and revised in relation to changes in health-care "structure, financing and delivery" (ANA, 2015a).

With nine provisions and associated interpretive statements, the code "restates the fundamental values and commitments of the nurse (Provisions 1–3), identifies the boundaries of duty and loyalty (Provisions 4–6), and describes the duties of the nurse that extend beyond individual patient encounters (Provisions 7–9)" (ANA, 2015a).

CODE OF ETHICS (ANA, 2015)	DISCUSSION
Provision 1. The nurse practices with compassion and respect for the inherent dignity, worth, and unique attributes of every person.	**The nurse respects all individuals in regard to dealings in care and communication. Nurses must abide by professional guidelines in all communication and in working with colleagues, patients and families. All individuals have the right to participate in their care**

"Code of Ethics for Nurses with Interpretive Statements," p. v. Copyright © 2015 by American Nurses Association.

Provision 2. The nurse's primary commitment is to the patient, whether an individual, family, group, community, or population.	**The nurse recognizes the need to include patients' input into their care. Conflicts of interest should be shared and addressed to avoid impacting patient care. Collaboration with others fosters best patient care. Consider the importance of professional boundaries and their relationship to patient care outcomes.**
Provision 3. The nurse promotes, advocates for, protects the rights, health, and safety of the patient.	**The nurse must understand all privacy guidelines related to patient care and patient identifiers. Nurses involved in research must understand all aspects of patient participation, including informed consent and full disclosure. The nurse is aware of institutional standards in place for performance review. Competence must be demonstrated in clinical and documentation skills. If there are questionable healthcare practice concerns, the nurse protects the patient by reporting misconduct.**
Provision 4. The nurse has authority, accountability, and responsibility for nursing practice; makes decisions; and takes action consistent with the obligation to provide optimal patient care.	**The nurse demonstrates accountability with responsible decision making regarding ethical concerns. Nursing decisions are well thought, planned, and purposefully implemented responsibly. Delegation of nursing activities is performed with respect for optimal results.**

Provision 5. The nurse owes the same duties to self as to others, including the responsibility to promote health and safety, preserve wholeness of character and integrity, maintain competence, and continue personal and professional growth	**The nurse demonstrates self-care, in addition to caring for others and implements safe practice from within the care setting extending to the community. Personal growth is demonstrated through lifelong learning.**
Provision 6. The nurse, through individual and collective effort, establishes, maintains, and improves the ethical environment of the work setting and conditions of employment that are conducive to safe, quality health care.	**As a nursing profession, standards should be outlined through all care environments regarding ethical obligations, including the need to report any safety, quality and environmental concerns that would negatively impact patient care outcomes.**
Provision 7. The nurse, in all roles and settings, advances the profession through research and scholarly inquiry, professional standards development, and the generation of both nursing and health policy.	**Nursing education includes principles of research, with informed application of scholarly work and inquiry into practice standards. Nursing organizations are encouraged to contribute to health policy and professional standards.**
Provision 8. The nurse collaborates with other health professionals and the public to protect human rights, promote health diplomacy, and reduce health disparities.	**Through collaboration within the discipline, and maintaining a practice philosophy that health is a right for all individuals, facilitates best practice standards. The nurse commits to lifelong learning through attendance at professional development activities.**
Provision 9. The profession of nursing, collectively through its professional organization, must articulate nursing values, maintain the integrity of the profession, and integrate principles of social justice into nursing and health policy.	**Participation on nursing committees and membership in professional organizations enables sharing of view and giving voice as an agent of change.**

FROM NOVICE TO EXPERT: BENNER'S STAGES OF CLINICAL COMPETENCE

A NURSE'S PERSPECTIVE

There are many things that can easily overwhelm new nurses ... in this case, a first code. My assigned patient was admitted with new onset of seizures. I was nervous but made sure to read all the reports and recommendations from the neurologist. I had just completed my rounds when the heart monitor at the desk alarmed. I ran into the room to see my patient experiencing a seizure. I called for help and calmly gave a report to the nursing staff about the patient while obtaining vital signs. A second later, the patient stopped breathing. The nurses on the unit assisted until the rapid response team (RRT) arrived with the physician. I suddenly froze and was unable to speak. I remember looking down at my hands vigorously shaking. Luckily, our unit's facilitator (resource) nurse was able to repeat my report during the code. The patient was given medications and eventually came out of a seizure that lasted a total of 8 minutes.

I "debriefed" with the nurse facilitator. As much as she tried to make me feel as though I did everything correctly, I felt discouraged because of the way I presented when the doctor and the team arrived. I remember her saying that I handled that situation calmly and cared for the patient professionally. She told me that I was able to report on the patient and the situation in a detailed, helpful way. I knew what the neurologist recommended, methods that worked for the patient, and applied this information. With time and more exposure to code situations, the facilitator said she was confident that those paralyzing nerves would disappear. *(RN to BS Student)*

Patricia Benner (1984) incorporated the Dreyfus model of skill acquisition when she published her research (**From Novice to Expert: Excellence and Power in Clinical Nursing Practice**). The accounts of experiences from practicing nurses enabled her to describe skill levels, in Stages 1 through 5, and articulate best practice learning techniques for each level. Benner believes that the most important way a nurse can enhance their practice is through experience. The stages outlined are crucial for the nurse to transition from novice to expert roles (Benner, 1984).

In **Stage 1, the novice (beginner)** has no experience in situations and expectations of performance. The novice requires repeated verbal and physical cues. Whether a beginner entering the profession or a veteran nurse changing specialties, the nurse will be expected to function in situations with no prior experience. With the experience gained from patient care, the novice develops skills for working through actual situations.

The advanced beginner, Stage 2, demonstrates marginally acceptable performance from experience in actual situations. The nurse in this stage is efficient and skillful in certain practice areas, yet needs periodic support and prompting. Advanced beginners have sufficient experience to be able to gather and interpret subjective and objective data. Advanced beginners rely on rules; however, with experience, they develop an awareness of additional characteristics that can be applied to related conditions.

The competent nurse of Stage 3 is employed in similar settings for more than 2 years. Competent nurses display efficiency, coordination, and confidence in their practice. They have become adept at planning, aiding in efficiency, and organizing. In planning care, the competent nurse incorporates both "conscious and abstract information," as well as "analytic contemplation of the situation" (Benner, 1984, p. 20). The outcome is enhanced efficiency, organization, and time management.

The proficient nurse (Stage 4) has been employed in the same or similar settings for three to five years. The proficient nurse considers situations in their entirety. With a holistic approach, proficient nurses anticipate which outcomes to expect in a particular situation and are able to modify the plan of care, respond efficiently and effectively to events, and meet the individualized needs of patients. In this stage, the proficient nurse demonstrates skill in the ability to prioritize problems and to make informed decisions.

Within **Stage 5, the expert nurse** possesses an instinctive understanding of each situation and demonstrates the ability to focus directly on the core of a problem. Examining each situation from a holistic viewpoint, the expert nurse's performance is informed, efficient, and organized. Highly skilled analytic ability is critical for new situations encountered and prevents precious time and energy expended on other findings. Years of experience contribute to the expert nurse's intuitive sense of the problem and skill needed for timely intervention.

A WORD ABOUT WRITING SKILLS

Hard writing makes easy reading.

~An old adage

In 2013, the ANA reported that communication skills are key competencies for RNs in all areas of practice. The ANA competency model stated that nurses must be able to clearly articulate in writing multiple decisions, plans, and activities essential to current professional nursing practice. Carefully constructed, clear, well-organized **writing skills** enable nurses to effectively and efficiently communicate with patients, families, and other members of the health-care team.

As nurses expand their careers, particularly if enrolled in advanced education programs, they must also learn how to compose journal articles, literature reviews, research papers, and dissertations. Also, nurses in current practice are continually encouraged to write about the fine work they carry out daily by publishing research findings in professional literature. However, beyond producing scholarly work for publication, nurses need writing skills daily to convey to the administration the need to generate scholarly projects, to obtain funding for necessary equipment and technology, and to achieve informed, positive change for professional practice and their respective health-care organization employers.

Johnson and Rulo (2019) examined the critical role of writing in nursing. In their presentation of a 10-point strategy for improving nurses' writing ability, they urged that good writing skills are "essential for the future of the nursing profession" (p. 57). Of the 10-point strategy, number six recommends that writers "consider the beginning and ending of your article." The beginning sets the pace for the entire essay, engages readers, and frames the argument. With a strong introduction, readers will look forward to consuming the article.

Johnson and Rulo (2019) urged nursing faculty to incorporate specific writing exercises into courses within the existing nursing curriculum. They encouraged working with the administration in higher education to create writing centers and employ writing coaches for students. In addition, sending timely feedback on edits and draft revisions can maximize student understanding and ultimately improve subsequent submissions. In evaluating student work, the authors stressed the use of specific rubrics introduced to students early on in the course as a valuable guideline in the practice and refinement of writing skills.

CHAPTER SUMMARY

In Chapter 1, the reader is afforded the opportunity to reflect on current practice and to examine the evidence related to returning to academia for an advanced degree. With the current climate in health care, it is vital that nurses equip themselves with the necessary education, experience, and expertise to strategize ways to meet those challenges head-on. Reflecting on nursing theorist Patricia Benner's *Novice to Expert* stages challenges the diverse population of ADN to BSN student readers (neophytes in professional nursing practice, practicing clinicians contemplating a change in nursing roles, veteran nurses seeking leadership and management positions) to begin to strategize and formulate goals for charting their future courses. The review of *Professional Practice Standards* supports the rationale for possessing an evidence-based practice philosophy, for maintaining professional development coupled with a code of integrity and caring, and for confirming the belief that lifelong learning in the nursing profession is essential. To this end, the reader is reminded of the importance of membership in professional nursing organizations to provide quality, informed care. Concurrently, evidence provided in Chapter 1 assists the reader with recognizing the need to refine writing skills to transform knowledge to practice and to ultimately achieve positive changes in the health-care setting.

FOOD FOR THOUGHT: CRITICAL THINKING QUESTIONS

1. After reading the ANA Standards and the Code of Ethics, how might you create your own definition of professionalism, accountability, responsibility, and civility?
2. As an RN returning to school for a baccalaureate degree in nursing, reading the description of Benner's novice to expert work, where do you believe you "fit"? Where would you place yourself within this five-stage model? Can you identify a similar process during your beginning practice as an RN? Why/why not?
3. Do nurses return to the novice stage with a new position/role change, or do they move in and out of different stages with role change or a new position? Give a reason and/or example for your responses.
4. Are the time frames for completion of each Benner stage realistic? Why/why not? How might you modify the length of time for each stage?
5. At what point (stage) do you think intuition (the ability to understand something immediately without the need for conscious reasoning) occurs?

SCENARIOS: APPLYING WHAT YOU HAVE LEARNED

Role Transition and Professional Responsibility

A recent BSN graduate who completed hospital-wide and unit orientation last month, Mark, works 32 hours (evenings) on a 20-bed adult surgical unit. He was previously employed on this same unit as a licensed practical nurse (LPN) for more than 5 years. Upon receiving his assignment tonight, Mark learns that he will be responsible ("charge") for the clients on half of the unit, which has a current census of 12 clients. His team consists of one LPN, a new ADN graduate who is still on orientation, two certified nursing assistants, and a unit secretary. Mark receives reports on the 12 clients: five new postoperative clients, two of whom are experiencing nausea and vomiting; two clients scheduled for surgery within the hour; four elderly clients requiring assistance with activities of daily living; and one client, postoperative day two, at high risk for falls. The nursing supervisor calls to say that she is in the process of securing "extra help" for the unit tonight and expresses confidence in Mark's abilities and his experience as an LPN.

In planning the assignment, and as part of the delegation process, respond to the following questions:

1.   What questions does Mark have for his nursing supervisor?
2.   What does Mark need to know about his team members?
3.   How does Mark organize and prioritize the care of these clients?
4.   What should the assignment sheet look like?
5.   What should Mark's assignment look like?

NURSING JOURNAL: REFLECT ON YOUR PRACTICE WHILE HONING YOUR WRITING SKILLS

The Critical Incident

A critical incident is one where you believe your intervention made a difference in your practice, directly or indirectly. It could involve one or more of the following: an incident that went unusually well, an incident in which there was a breakdown (things didn't go as planned), an incident that is very ordinary, an incident that was particularly demanding, or an incident that captures the epitome of nursing.

1.   **Describe the critical incident** (context of the incident, resources available).
2.   **Give a detailed description of what happened** (why do you think the incident was "critical"?).
3.   **Discuss your concerns at the time** (what was particularly demanding/satisfying about the incident?).
4.   **Identify a nursing theorist with whom you relate** (and who perhaps affected your decision making at the time of the critical incident).

CHAPTER 1 REFERENCES

Aiken L. H., Clarke S. P., Cheung R. B., Sloane D. M., & Silber J. H. (2003). Educational levels of hospital nurses and surgical patient mortality. *Journal of the American Medical Association*, *290*(12), 1617–1623. http://doi.org/10.1001/jama.290.12.1617

American Association of Colleges of Nursing (AACN). (2008). *The essentials of baccalaureate education for professional nursing practice.* http://www.aacn.nche.edu/education-resources/baccessentials08.pdf

American Association of Colleges of Nursing (AACN). (2019a). 2018–2019 Enrollment and graduations in baccalaureate and graduate programs in nursing. https://www.aacnnursing.org/Portals/42/News/Factsheets/Faculty-Shortage-Factsheet.pdf

American Association of Colleges of Nursing. (2019b). AACN Fact sheet 2018–2019.

American Nurses Association. (ANA). (2001a). *Code of ethics for nurses with interpretive statements.* Nurses Books.

American Nurses Association. (ANA). (2014c). *Code of ethics for nurses with interpretive statements.* Nurses Books.

American Nurses Association. (ANA). (2015a). *Code of ethics for nurses with interpretive statements.* Nurses Books.

American Nurses Association. (ANA). (2015b). *Nursing: Scope and standards of practice* (3rd ed.).

Anbari A. B. (2015). The RN to BSN transition: A qualitative systematic review. *Global Qualitative Nursing Research, 2.* http://doi.org/10.1177/2333393615614306

Benner, P. (1984). *From novice to expert, excellence and power in clinical nursing practice.* Addison-Wesley Publishing Company.

Buerhaus, P., Skinner, L., Auerbach, D. & Stager, D. (2017). Four challenges facing the nursing work force in the United States. *Journal of Nursing Regulation, 8*(2). https://doi.org/10.1016/s2155-8256(18) 30015-2

Catallo, C., Spalding, K., & Haghiri-Vijeh, R. (2014). Nursing professional organizations: What are they doing to engage nurses in health policy? *Sage Open, 4*(4), 1–9. https://doi.org/10.1177/2158244014560534

Clifford, M. E., & Jurado, L. F. (2018). The impact of an all BSN workforce policy. *Journal of Nursing Practice Applications & Reviews of Research, 8*(2), 60–67.

Davis, C. (2014). The importance of professional standards. *Nursing Made Incredibly Easy, 1.* http://doi.org/10.1097/01.NME.0000452691.04516.96

Haddad, L. M., & Toney-Butler, T. J. (2019). *Nursing shortage.* StatPearls Publishing. https://www.ncbi.nlm.nih.gov/books/NBK493175/

Halter, M., Boiko, O., Pelone, F., Beighton, C., Harris, R., Gale, R., Gourlay, S., & Drennan, V. (2017). The determinants and consequences of adult nursing staff turnover: A systematic review of systematic reviews. *BMC Health Services Research, 17*(824), 1–20. https://doi.org/10.1186/s12913-017-2707-0

Institute of Medicine (IOM). (2010). *The future of nursing: Leading change, advancing health.* National Academies Press.

Johnson, J., & Rulo, K. (2019). Problem in the profession: How and why writing skills in nursing must be improved. *Journal of Professional Nursing, 35*(2019), 57–64.

Matthews, J. (2012). Role of professional organizations in advocating for the nursing profession. *OJIN: The Online Journal of Issues in Nursing 17*(1). https://doi.org/10.3912/OJIN.Vol17No01Man03

Osterman P. L., Asselin M. E., & Cullen, H. A. (2009). Returning for a baccalaureate: A descriptive exploratory study of nurses' perceptions. *Journal for Nurses in Staff Development (JNSD), 25*, 109–117. https://doi.org/10.1097/NND.0b013e3181a566be

Perfetto, L. M. (2015). Facilitating educational advancement of RNs to the baccalaureate: What are they telling us? *Nursing Education Perspectives, 36*(1), 34–41. https://doi.org/10.5480/13-1161.1

Romp, C., Kiehl, E., Bickett, A., Bledsoe, S., Brown, D., Eitel, S., & Wall, M. (2014). Motivators and barriers to returning to school: RN to BSN (2014). *Journal for Nurses in Professional Development, 30*(2), 83–86.

Roux, G., & Halstead, J. (2018). *Issues and trends in nursing, practice, policy and leadership* (2nd ed.), Jones and Bartlett Learning.

Slattery M., Logan B., Mudge, B., Secore K., von Reyn L., & Maue, R. (2016). An undergraduate research fellowship program to prepare nursing students for future workforce roles. *Journal of Professional Nursing, 32*(6), 412–420.

OTHER RESOURCES

https://www.bls.gov/ooh/healthcare/registered-nurses.htm

http://www.nln.org/docs/default-source/newsroom/nursing-education-statistics/percentage-of-students-over-age-30-by-program-type-2014.pdf?sfvrsn=0

https://www.aacnnursing.org/Nursing-Education-Programs/Baccalaureate-Education

https://onlinelearningconsortium.org/read/digital-learning-compass-distance-education-enrollment-report-2017/

Disseminate Knowledge and Caring

CHAPTER INTRODUCTION

The content in this chapter highlights the importance of adopting and disseminating a "knowledge and caring" philosophy for professional nursing practice. These concepts echo Florence Nightingale's endorsement of the "the art and science" of nursing, coupling evidence with empathy to effect positive change in the care of patients, families, and communities (Nightingale,1992). As an extension of Chapter 1, Chapter 2 expands upon the Code of Ethics in Nursing provisions as they relate to caring behaviors, foundational ethical principles, civil behaviors, and healthy practice environments.

KEY TERMS: MAKING CONNECTIONS

- Autonomy
- Beneficence
- Caring
- Change agent
- Cognitive rehearsal
- Ethics and civility
- Ethical decision making
- Justice
  - Distributive
  - Social
- Nonmaleficence

LEARNING OBJECTIVES/OUTCOMES

In this chapter, students will accomplish the following:

- Discuss methods of conducting and translating research into clinical practice.
- Explain the meaning of the knowledge-caring dyad.
- Describe strategies to create a civil environment in both clinical and academic settings.
- Apply ethical and professional standards when developing an evidence-based plan of care.

Care is the essence of nursing and the central, dominant, and unifying focus of nursing

—*Madeleine Leininger*

Caring may occur without curing but curing cannot occur without caring.

—*Jean Watson*

A NURSE'S PERSPECTIVE

Jean Watson's theory on the philosophy of care has long fascinated me. Her Theory of Human Caring/Caring Science is based on the idea that we as nurses can be healers by showing kindness and meeting the needs of our patients not purely through the physical aspects of care, but also the emotional and spiritual aspects. We as nurses are to be "authentically present" for our patients. Watson discusses the need for nurses to search their own beliefs and take care of their own emotional and spiritual needs. Her theory even allows for the possibility of miracles (Watson, 2008). I was struck by her theory because it aligns so closely with how I wish to conduct my nursing practice. (RN-BS student)

DISSEMINATE KNOWLEDGE

With more nurses working in the health-care trenches than any other health-care profession, nursing research is increasingly recognized as a critical pathway to developing realistic methods to reduce hospital errors and unnecessary costs (World Health Organization, 2012). As such, nurse-led research is increasingly recognized as a critical pathway to practical and effective ways of improving patient outcomes. However, there are barriers to the translation of research evidence into practice that must be addressed and resolved (Curtis et al., 2016).

There is general agreement that patient care should be based on the best available evidence (ANA, 2015a; ANA, 2015b). Knowledge and evidence received from sound quality scholarly methods should guide nurses' clinical practice and care decisions to effect change. Conveying research evidence to clinical practice is crucial for delivering safe, transparent, and efficient health care to meet the needs of patients, families, and the community.

RESEARCH TRANSLATION BARRIERS

Competing priorities in the health-care setting can challenge attempts to introduce and integrate evidence as a means of improving delivery of patient care. Successful implementation of research evidence into clinical practice is dependent on changing human behavior. Any attempt to improve the quality of care for patients by introducing research must incorporate a clear understanding of the associated barriers to, and facilitators of, behavior change. Such barriers may involve clinician behavior, time elements for developing evidence-based guidelines, scarcity of continuing education programs, lack of administrative support, and resistant organizational culture. Understanding these barriers is fundamental to the development of a feasible, successful implementation strategy (Wallis, 2012).

Disseminating best practices can lead to transparent, sustainable health-care delivery. Successful interpretation and incorporation of research data has the potential to affect cultural, behavioral, and practical change, thereby reducing the research-practice gap. Research findings must be translated early on in the change process, starting with research design, to obtaining the feedback of end users in the evaluation process. The attainment of research implementation ultimately depends on behavior change. It is critical that the implementation strategy include this element (Wallis, 2012).

DISSEMINATING RESEARCH KNOWLEDGE

Crucial to nurse-led research and knowledge, translation is the distribution of information. A research study is not complete until the study findings have been translated via presentations at professional forums and published in a peer-reviewed publication. It is here where appropriate recommendations are made regarding how the research findings could be integrated into nursing practice. Opportunities for sharing research outcomes and new knowledge can be realized through social media, public speaking events, "lunch and learn" seminars, and poster presentations.

The success of research implementation in health care is dependent on clinician/consumer behavior change. The success of this outcome is largely dependent on how findings will be circulated, a consideration to be included early on in the research planning stages. Those interested in publicizing their findings must be cognizant of this element throughout the research implementation process.

DISSEMINATING CARING

Caring is a universal human attribute that has endured the test of time. Caring is integral to the profession of nursing as the very foundation upon which the underpinnings of nursing practice are grounded. Complexities of patient care, nursing workloads, and advanced technologies have changed significantly since Nightingale's time, thus challenging the practice and genuineness of caring. However, caring remains at the core of the art and science of nursing practice, despite some perceived fears of its loss (Adams, 2016).

Nurses learn how best to develop their ability to "walk a mile in another's shoes." This ensures that those individuals who work with vulnerable populations have an attitude that enables them to empathize, listen to, and learn from others' experiences (Hemingway, 2013). Evidence clarifies that caring and empathy in nursing positively affect clinical nursing practice. Sumner (2005) reported that while nurses today require a higher level of skill and knowledge for technologically advanced machinery and tests, a "hands-on" caring approach is irreplaceable.

In a meta-analysis of 130 studies published between 1980 and 1996, Swanson (1999) reported the outcomes of **caring** for patients and nurses. Positive outcomes for **patients** included emotional-spiritual (positive self-esteem, knowledge, and coping), physical (improved healing), and social (trust) results. Positive outcomes for **nurses** included emotional-spiritual (sense of accomplishment, self-satisfaction, fulfillment), professional (such as increased skills and knowledge, satisfaction with nursing), and social (as in enhanced relationships with patients).

Caring beliefs may vary, but their meanings are the same. Caring, according to Watson (2008), requires personal, social, moral, and spiritual engagement of the nurse, as well as a commitment to self and others. To truly care is to be compassionate; otherwise, nurses are carrying out interventions in a detached state. Removal of the nurturing factor may not necessarily alter the performance of nursing actions, but the overall healing process may actually change (Nelson & Watson, 2011).

Improving the experiences and satisfaction of patients and caregivers has been a high priority in achieving quality care (Adams, 2016; Schearer, 2015; Sumner, 2005; Swanson, 1999; Watson, 2008). The production of high-quality care requires health-care providers to be competent, responsible, and empathetic. The care of patients and families entails not only diagnosing and treating patients' physical illnesses but also caring for their hearts and souls. In exercising a "head" (cognitive), "heart" (affective), and "hands (psychomotor) approach, providers support the holistic needs of patients, foster compliance with treatment, and achieve desired patient outcomes.

For the nursing profession, recognizing gaps between the mission and values of practice organizations in the delivery of care is critical. We must recognize, acknowledge, and act upon those gaps. In the debriefing process, in reviewing occurrences when care has diverged from anticipated outcomes, transparency in acknowledging errors can restore purpose.

CLINICAL SIGNIFICANCE OF THE CODE OF ETHICS

The term **ethics** is derived from the Greek *ethos*, or character. Ethics are moral principles that govern how a person or group will behave or conduct themselves (Östman etal., 2019). Nurses face ethical dilemmas regularly and make sound decisions based on their values, supported by the laws that govern them.

For informed, competent practice, nurses are guided by the ANA's Code of Ethics (American Nurses Association [ANA], 2015a). This important work provides a concise statement regarding the ethical responsibilities of nurses. Revised over time, the current version of the Code includes technological developments, workplace environments, societal changes, advanced practice roles, research, education, and health policy (Epstein & Turner, 2015).

Refer to Chapter 1 to view the nine provisions of the Code of Ethics with descriptions.

ETHICAL DILEMMAS

Ethical dilemmas surface as nurses care for patients. These dilemmas may conflict with both the Code of Ethics and with the nurse's values. As patient advocates, nurses need to find a midpoint in the provision of care. To find this midpoint, nurses rely on four main principles of ethics: (1) **autonomy** (independence), (2) **beneficence** (promote only good), (3) **justice** (fairness), and (4) **nonmaleficence** (do no harm). (Östman et al., 2019). Other important principles in ethical decision making include veracity, advocacy, caring, and confidentiality (Koloroutis & Thorstenson, 1999).

Autonomy is the ethical principle by which patients have the right to make independent decisions based on their own beliefs and values (Beauchamp & Childress, 2001). A patient's need for autonomy may conflict with guidelines that nurses or other health-care workers believe are best. The patient has a right to refuse medications, treatment, surgery, or other medical interventions. If a patient declines a treatment deemed beneficial, the nurse must acknowledge that decision (Östman et al., 2019).

The concept of **nonmaleficence** informs nurses to "do no harm," either intentionally or unintentionally, to patients (Beauchamp & Childress, 2001). The obligation here is not only to prevent harm but also to prevent exposing the patient to a "harmful" risk. With **beneficence**, nurses must abstain from maltreatment, minimize harm, and promote goodwill toward patients. This principle is demonstrated by providing a balance of "benefits against risks" to patients. Examples where nurses apply beneficence in their practice include assisting patients with activities that they cannot carry out independently, instituting fall precautions, and administering medications safely (Östman et al., 2019).

As an obligation to maintain impartiality to all individuals, the ethical principle of **justice** encompasses fairness and equality (Beauchamp & Childress, 2001). With **distributive justice**, individuals have the right to be treated equally regardless of ethnic group, gender, culture, age, marital status, medical diagnosis, social standing, economic level, or political or religious beliefs; whereas **social justice** is based on access to equal rights, regardless of one's individual characteristics (Östman et al., 2019). Nurses employ distributive and social justice with patients by enabling them to exercise their rights through inclusion and empowerment.

Nurses are challenged to identify and act upon ethical issues that affect them, their colleagues, and their patients. Equally important is the need for health-care organizations to have available current, appropriate, and professional resources to resolve ethical dilemmas. Hospital organizations engage multidisciplinary ethics committees whose members meet as a group to resolve ethical dilemmas and conflicts. There should be at least one nurse on such a committee. Outcomes of all interventions to foster ethical practice should be evaluated and measured. Evaluation criteria of such outcomes should consider knowledge of ethics and ethical dilemmas in daily practice. Patients should be evaluated regarding their awareness of ethical practices in their health-care organization, as well as their rights as consumers of care (ANA, 2015a; ANA, 2015b; Epstein & Turner, 2015; Koloroutis & Thorstenson, 1999).

ETHICS AND CIVILITY IN NURSING

THROUGH A STUDENT LENS: A PERSPECTIVE ON INCIVILITY

Throughout my clinical rotations, I was struck by the environmental toxicity that can fester between nurses. Typically, a miscommunication would trigger animosity and the toxicity would be fueled by different groups of nurses circling their wagons to defend their point of view.

As a student and impartial observer, I could see this play out between different shifts of nurses on the same floor, and also between floors if the work required many patient transfers within the hospital. This issue is important to me because I saw first-hand how it negatively impacts morale, increases stress, and has the potential to negatively impact patient care. In their work, Wei et al. (2018) concluded, "The key to ensuring patients' quality of care is a healthy work environment, which is essential in promoting nurse satisfaction, retention, and performance" (p. 298). Achieving that healthy work environment would be a priority for me if I ever found myself in a leadership role, one most certainly predicated on obtaining a BSN.

I rotated frequently among these groups and gained insight by seeing the root of a grievance from all sides. I could see that the ED was not "careless," the night shift was not "lazy," the ICU was not "demanding." They were all skilled nurses doing their best given their unique set of circumstances. My brief exposure in all settings helped develop empathy for the different challenges faced by all groups of nurses. It led me to believe that if all nurses were given the opportunity to rotate through groups they interact with regularly, interpersonal relationships would improve. Cultivating interpersonal relationships would foster effective communication strategies, improve both morale and retention, and have the positive impact on patient care predicted by Wei et al. (2018). (RN to BS student)

For the 18th year in a row, Americans rate the honesty and ethics of nurses as highest when compared among a list of professions that Gallup asks U.S. citizens to evaluate each year (Gallup, 2020). Currently, 85% of Americans say nurses' honesty and ethical standards are "very high" or "high." An 84% finding was reported in 2018. The nursing profession is regularly rated higher in honesty and ethics than all other professions, according to Gallup survey results.

Clark (2017) encouraged nurses to continue their vigilance in maintaining this distinction. The Code of Ethics for Nurses with Interpretive Statements (ANA, 2015a) clearly communicates the profession's responsibility to promote respectful safe, ethical, and civil workplaces. Nurses are obliged to "create an ethical environment and culture of civility and kindness, treating colleagues, coworkers, employees, students, and others with dignity and respect and that any form of bullying, harassment, intimidation, manipulation, threats or violence will not be tolerated" (ANA, 2015a, p. 4).

Incivility and bullying are part of a "constellation of harmful actions taken and those not taken" in the workplace (Saltzberg, 2011, p. 229). This definition provides a comprehensive explanation that includes using obvious displays of uncivil or threatening acts. Also, the definition includes a failure to respond when action is necessary or required to address workplace incivility, bullying, or violence. As a significant issue among health-care providers in health-care settings (Christie & Jones, 2013; Clark, 2017; Clark & Ahten,

2014; Clark & Springer, 2007), incivility disrupts social norms, lowers morale, decreases productivity, and, ultimately, negatively affects the well-being of both patient and nurse.

Rocker (2012) suggested that increased workloads and the ever-changing structure of health-care organizations are major contributing factors to uncivil behavior. Reactions to increased stress in the workplace are often demonstrated by transferring these frustrations to others, typically subordinates, such as novice nurses or new employees (Christie & Jones, 2013). There may exist an "eat their young" attitude in the workplace culture, conveying a message that new graduates must tolerate this incivility as they "prove" their worth (Longo, 2013). Moreover, "veteran nurses" in this setting may not be equipped with the conflict resolution skills or administrative support needed to defend those individuals being harassed (Vessey et al., 2009).

Uncivil behavior can add to nurses' stress load when they are already overburdened in a demanding work setting (Blair, 2013; Christie & Jones, 2013). Incivility can also cause a breakdown in staff's collaborative relationships (Longo, 2013; Rosenstein, 2011). Additional research reports higher institutional operating expenses because of staff absenteeism and turnover, as well as staff replacement and mediation costs— secondary outcomes of uncivil behavior (Blair, 2013; Luparello, 2011; Rocker, 2012).

Lim and Bernstein (2014) described individual and system factors that contributed to incivility in the workplace. Individual factors cited included self-centeredness, immaturity, defensiveness, and lack of conflict management skills. System factors involved job pressure, empowerment roles, and continual changes related to shift rotations (Lim & Bernstein, 2014).

Decreased communication as a result of negative behaviors lowers morale and interferes with effective dialog, critical thinking, and decision making for nurses (Blair, 2013). A lack of communication leads to lowered productivity and, ultimately, affects the working environment, thus risking the quality of care delivered and culminating in adverse events, which compromise the overall safety for both nurses and patients.

Growing evidence validates the importance of reciprocal relationships between healthy work environments and optimal patient outcomes. Nurses employed in unhealthy settings work in an environment of lowered quality of patient care, often with an inferior hospital reputation (Wei et al., 2018). Unhealthy work environments are linked to higher occurrences of hospital-acquired conditions, patient mortality, failure to rescue, and readmission rates and contribute to staff dissatisfaction, low morale, and high turnover (Buhlman, 2016; Lasater & McHugh, 2016; McHugh & Ma, 2016).

Following a comprehensive examination of the work environments where critical care nurses practice, the American Association of Critical-Care Nurses (AACN, 2005) advocated for settings that promote excellence in patient care and support all members of the health-care team in experiencing fulfillment from their work. The *Standards for*

Establishing and Sustaining Healthy Work Environments: A Journey to Excellence (2005) outlined six essential standards for healthy work environments: (1) skilled communication, (2) true collaboration, (3) effective decision making, (4) appropriate staffing, (5) meaningful recognition, and (6) authentic leadership.

A second edition of the AACN standards (2016) supported the ongoing significance and continuation of the six standards, confirming a crucial link between healthy work environments and optimal outcomes for patients, health-care professionals, and health-care organizations. The AACN healthy work environment standards and their associated critical elements are a "blueprint" that assists nursing, other health-care providers, and administrators in creating and maintaining best practices (AACN, 2016).

A proactive, collaborative approach is essential to fostering civility in the workplace. Leaders in health care can encourage civility among nursing staff by first establishing a zero-tolerance policy for violence. Staff must be educated on how to recognize the potential for violence, how to employ de-escalation techniques, and how to seek assistance to prevent or respond to violence. A foundational structure for workplace violence must be in place, with specific policies and procedures on how to report violent incidents to law enforcement.

In recognizing triggers for uncivil behavior, nurse managers and administrators must evaluate staffing patterns as well as patient classification systems, both of which have the potential to affect violent events. Concurrently, quality security systems must be in place, including alarms, emergency response, sufficient staffing, and the steady presence of security personnel. In addition, providing staff education and counseling programs upon orientation to the position with annual in-service programs will empower nurses to anticipate and to manage escalating disruptive or inappropriate behaviors.

Cognitive rehearsal (CR) (Clark, 2017; Griffin & Clark, 2014) is an evidence-based technique used to help individuals deal with potentially stressful conflict through rehearsing ways to address the situation with the hope of achieving a favorable outcome. Being well-prepared, speaking with confidence, and using respectful language to address incivility serve to empower nurses and other health-care professionals to advocate for patient safety and workplace health. CR prepares people for uncivil encounters through the steps of prebriefing, identifying scenarios for simulation, role-playing and rehearsing responses, practicing simulated scenarios repeatedly, and debriefing after the encounter.

A study by Hersch et al. (2016) sought to determine the effectiveness of a web-based stress management program designed specifically for nurses and the conflict situations they may face. The *BREATHE: Stress Management for Nurses* program was designed to provide nurses with the means to manage stressors that affect their practice. This web-based process affords nurses access to the program at times that are convenient for their daily personal and professional schedules and provides them with the opportunity to progress through the program at their own pace.

The *BREATHE* program consists of six comprehensive modules (and an additional module for nurse managers): (1) "Welcome and Introduction," (2) "Assess Your Stress," (3) "Identify Stressors," (4) "Manage Stress," (5) "Avoid Negative Coping, and (6) "Your Mental Health." The manager's role includes additional education for nurse leaders. The additional module is designed to help managers identify and address potential workplace stressors. With this education, leaders are able to anticipate and reduce stress through positive management practices (Hersch et al., 2016).

Experimental group participants were encouraged to use *BREATHE* as often as was necessary over a 3-month period. Included in the program was the Nursing Stress Scale (NSS), which assessed seven sources of work-related stress (Gray-Toft & Anderson, 1981). Subscales of this measure include death and dying, conflict with physicians, inadequate preparation, lack of support, conflict with other nurses, workload, and uncertainty concerning treatment. The NSS scores on each of the seven subscales, as well as the total stress score, measure the frequency with which the seven major sources of nursing stress are experienced by the participant (Hersch et al., 2016).

Overall, study findings indicated that the *BREATHE* web-based program was an effective means of reducing nurses' perceived stress related to the subscale issues cited earlier (Hersch et al., 2016). Results of the study give hope for the use of web-based programs as important occupationally based interventions to help nurses gain the needed information and skills to manage stressors associated with nursing that can trigger instances of incivility.

CHAPTER SUMMARY

Nurses cannot practice safely, professionally, and skillfully without a foundation of current, quality evidence to support sound, informed interventions. In Chapter 2, the reader is presented with the concepts of knowledge and caring as foundational building blocks in creating change. As powerful as experience, education, and expertise are for the nurse, translating that knowledge into practice is equally valued. Research translation requires intelligence, caring, empathy, and patience when encouraging others to integrate new evidence-based findings into their practice.

The stability of the workplace environment, timing of changes to be made, staff acceptance, and readiness of the administration to acknowledge and participate in the change process are major factors to consider when presenting new ideas. More than likely, these influences will converge to test the civility of participants and threaten progress.

In this chapter, readers were reminded of the impact of ethics and the application of ethical principles as major tenets of professional nursing practice. Ethical dilemmas touch nurse's lives daily. In particular, baccalaureate graduates, as future leaders and decision makers, must possess, value, and apply these principles in all aspects of critical thinking and decision making.

FOOD FOR THOUGHT: CRITICAL THINKING QUESTIONS

1. Where do the topics of incivility, lateral violence, and bullying belong in the nursing education curriculum?
2. What experiences have you had with conflict resolution (skills needed, obstacles, challenges, successes, impact)?
3. How are nurses' ethical principles integrated into patients' care plans? Create a discharge plan for your patient that includes three of the principles in this chapter.
4. What is the difference between distributive justice and social justice? Give an example of each as it relates to health care.

SCENARIO: APPLYING WHAT YOU HAVE LEARNED

Incivility

With a track record of positive reviews and a recognized future leader by all who work with her, Rachel was promoted to the role of nurse manager of a 40-bed medical unit 3 months ago. She has worked on this unit since graduation from LPN school, returned for her ADN 5 years ago, and last year received her baccalaureate degree in nursing. Because of a recent reorganization, the hospital has experienced a change in the nursing administration. Rachel's current supervisor's approach contradicts both her democratic leadership style and the philosophy of her mentor, a supportive leader who has left the organization for a high-level nursing management position in another city. Rachel has found the new supervisor to be authoritative and negative. When Rachel has attempted to discuss unit issues with her, her supervisor has replied that she was "too busy" and that Rachel "needed to develop a backbone." Yesterday, the supervisor told Rachel that she must fire an outspoken nurse—an industrious, well-respected staff member with more than 20 years at the organization—who had been openly expressing his frustration with the hospital's reorganization plan and the resultant disorganization on the unit.

1. As nurse manager, what is Rachel's next step?
2. If Rachel came to you, what advice would you give to her?
3. What questions would you ask?
4. What factors must be considered?

Support your response with an actual plan; describe the series of events that you would like to see unfold for a resolution of this situation.

NURSING JOURNAL: REFLECT ON YOUR PRACTICE WHILE HONING YOUR WRITING SKILLS

Ethics

A 28-year old mother of three children (9, 5, and 2 years) is admitted to the hospital's surgical unit from the emergency department with symptoms of epigastric pain, nausea, and vomiting of 2-day duration. Diagnostic tests reveal acute cholecystitis. She is scheduled for laparoscopic cholecystectomy.

During the admission assessment, the patient expresses concern about her partner's ability to care for her children. She also appears worried about how she will manage at home after she is discharged. The nurse offers to contact the client's husband. In addition, she places a request for a social service consult, suggests a family meeting, and informs the patient that visiting nursing services can be arranged.

What assumptions on the part of the nurse are being made here? Using the ethical principles of beneficence, maleficence, autonomy, and justice, how might the nurse better assess and intervene in this situation?

Assumptions
Ethical Principles

    a. Autonomy
    b. Beneficence
    c. Maleficence
    d. Justice

CHAPTER 2 REFERENCES

Adams, L. (2016). The conundrum of caring in nursing. *International Journal of Caring Sciences,* 9(1),1–8.

American Association of Critical-Care Nurses (AACN). (2005). *AACN standards for establishing and sustaining healthy work environments: A journey to excellence.*

American Association of Critical-Care Nurses (AACN). (2016). *AACN standards for establishing and sustaining healthy work environments: A journey to excellence* (2nd ed.).

American Nurses Association. (ANA). (2015a) *Code of ethics for nurses, with interpretive statements.*

American Nurses Association. (ANA). (2015b). *Nursing: Scope and standards of practice* (3rd ed.).

American Nurses Association. (2015). *Professional issues panel on incivility, bullying, and workplace violence. Position statement on incivility, bullying, and workplace violence.* www.nursingworld.org/Policy-Advocacy/Positions-and-Resolutions/ANAPositionStatements/Position-Statements-Alphabetically/IncivilityBullying-and-Workplace-Violence.html

Beauchamp, T., & Childress, J. (2001). *Principles of biomedical ethics.* Oxford University Press.

Blair, P. (2013). Lateral violence in nursing. *Journal of Emergency Nursing, 39*(5), e75–78.

Buhlman, N. (2016). How nurses' work environment influences key performance indicators. *American Nurse Today, 11*(3), 54–56.

Christie, W., & Jones, S. (2013). Lateral violence in nursing and the theory of the nurse as wounded healer. *OJIN: The Online Journal of Issues in Nursing, 19*(1). https://doi.org/10.3912/OJIN.Vol19NO01PPT01

Clark, C. (2017). Fostering a culture of civility and respect in nursing. *Journal of Nursing Regulation, 10*(1), 44–52.

Clark, C., & Springer, P. (2007) Incivility in nursing education: A descriptive study of definitions and prevalence. *Journal of Nursing Education, 46* (1), 7–14.

Clark, C., Ahten, S., & Macy, R. (2014). Nursing graduates' ability to address incivility: Kirkpatrick's level-3 evaluation. *Clinical Simulation in Nursing, 10*(8), 425–443.

Curtis, K., Fry, M., Shaban, R., & Considine, J. (2016). Translating research findings to clinical nursing practice. *Journal of Clinical Nursing, 26*, 862–872. https://10.1111/jocn.13586

Epstein, B., & Turner, M. (2015). The nursing code of ethics: Its value, its history. *OJIN: The Online Journal of Issues in Nursing, 20*(2), Manuscript 4.

Gallup Poll. (2020). Honesty/ethics in professions. Retrieved January 31, 2020, from http://www.gallup.com/poll/1654/honesty-ethicsprofessions.aspx.

Gray-Toft, P., & Anderson J. (1981) The nursing stress scale: Development of an instrument. *Journal of Behavioral Assessment, 3*(1), 11–23.

Griffin, M., & Clark, C. (2014). Revisiting cognitive rehearsal as an intervention against incivility and lateral violence in nursing: 10 years later. *Journal of Continuing Education in Nursing, 45*(12), 535–544.

Hemingway, A. (2013). What is nursing care and who owns it? *Nursing Times.* https://www.nursingtimes.net/roles/nurse-managers/what-is-nursing-care-and-who-owns-it-05-02-2013/

Hersch, R., Royer, F., Cook, K., Deitz, S., Kaplan, D., Hughes, M., Fries, M., &Vezina, M. (2016). Reducing nurses' stress: A randomized controlled trial of a web-based stress management program for nurses. *Applied Nursing Research, 32*, 18–25. https://doi.org/10.1016/j.apnr.2016.04.003.

Koloroutis, M., & Thorstenson, T. (1999). An ethics framework for organizational change. *Nursing Administrative Quarterly, 23*(2), 9–18.

Lasater, K. B., & McHugh, M. D. (2016). Nurse staffing and the work environment linked to read-missions among older adults following elective total hip and knee replacement. *International Journal for Quality in Health Care, 28*(2), 253–258.

Lim, F., & Bernstein, I. (2014). Civility and workplace bullying: Resonance of Nightingale's persona and current best practices. *Nursing Forum, 49*(2), 124–129.

Longo, J. (2013). Combating disruptive behaviors: Strategies to promote a healthy work environment. *OJIN: The Online Journal of Issues in Nursing, 15*(1), Manuscript 5. https://doi.org/10.3912/OJIN.Vol15N001Man05

Luparell, S. (2011). Incivility in nursing: The connection between academia and clinical settings. *Critical Care Nurse, 31*(2), 92–95.

McHugh, M. D., & Ma, C. (2016). Wage, work environment, and staffing: Effects on nurse outcomes. *Policy, Politics, & Nursing Practice, 15*(3–4), 72–80.

Nelson, J., & Watson, J. (2011). *Measuring caring: International research on caritas as healing.* Springer Publishing Company.

Nightingale F. Notes on nursing: What it is and what it is not. London: Lippincott Williams and Wilkins; 1992.

Östman, L., Näsman, Y., Eriksson, K., & Nyström, L. (2019). Ethos: The heart of ethics and health. *Nursing Ethics, 26*(1), 26–36. https://doi.org/10.1177/0969733017695655

Rocker, C. (2012). Responsibility of a frontline manager regarding staff bullying. *The Online Journal of Issues in Nursing, 18*(2). https://doi.org/10.3912/OJIN.Vol17NOO3PPTO2

Rosenstein, A. (2011). Managing disruptive behaviors in the health care setting: Focus on obstetrics services. *American Journal of Obstetrics and Gynecology, 204*(3), 187–192.

Saltzberg, C. W. (2011.) Balancing in moments of vulnerability while dancing the dialectic. *Advances in Nursing Science, 34*(3), 229–242.

Schearer, J. (2015). Critique of nursing as caring theory: Aesthetic knowing and caring in online learning. *International Journal for Human Caring, 19*(2), 45–49.

Sumner, J. (2005). Caring—the foundation of advanced practice nursing. *Topics in Advanced Practice Nursing, 4*(4), 12–16.

Swanson, K. (1999). Effects of caring, measurement, and time on miscarriage impact and women's well-being. *Nursing Research, 48*(6), 288–298.

Vessey, J., Demarco, R., Gaffney, D., & Budin, W. (2009). Bullying of staff registered nurses in the workplace: A preliminary study for developing personal and organizational strategies for the transformation of hostile to healthy workplace environments. *Journal of Professional Nursing, 25*(5), 299–306.

Wallis, L. (2012). Barriers to implementing evidence-based practice remain high for U.S. nurses. *American Journal of Nursing, 112*, 15.

Watson, J. (2008). *Nursing: The philosophy and science of caring.* University Press of Colorado.

Wei, H., Sewell, K. A., Woody, G., & Rose, M. A. (2018). The state of the science of nurse work environments in the United States: A systematic review. *International Journal of Nursing Sciences, 5*(3), 287–300.

World Health Organization. (2012). Enhancing nursing and midwifery capacity to contribute the prevention, treatment and management of noncommunicable diseases in practice: Policy and advocacy, research and education. *Human Resources for Health Observer, 12,* 1–32.

Provide Patient-Centered Care

CHAPTER INTRODUCTION

This chapter introduces the reader to the IOM's core competency of patient-centered care and the challenges health-care providers face to meet expected levels of achievement today. The origin of the term "patient-centered" care and related principles are explored.

The caring theories of Leininger, Orem, Peplau, and Watson are examined. Strategies for integrating patient culture, ethnicity, and social determinants of health when planning care are presented, along with an overview of current progress with the Healthy People 2020 goals.

KEY TERMS: MAKING CONNECTIONS

- Autonomy
- Culturally sensitive care
- Healthy People 2020
- Leininger's theory of culture care diversity and universality
- Orem's self-care theory
- Patient/person-centered care
- Peplau's interpersonal relations theory
- Picker's Eight Principles of Patient-Centered Care
- Quality and safety education in nursing (QSEN)
- Social determinants of health (SDH)
- Transparency
- Watson's Caring Theory

LEARNING OBJECTIVES/OUTCOMES

At the end of this chapter, students will accomplish the following:

- Recognize the origin and significance of "patient-centered care" principles.
- Identify strategies to fulfill the IOM patient-centered care competencies.
- Describe the caring theories of selected nursing theorists.
- Discuss the Healthy People 2020 national initiative.
- Explain the importance of culture and ethnicity when planning, providing, and evaluating patient care.

> Care is the essence of nursing and the central, dominant,
> and unifying focus of nursing.
>
> —*Madeleine Leininger*

A NURSE'S PERSPECTIVE

I was assigned to MB, an elderly Jordanian man whose primary language was Arabic, with some English, and a diagnosis of pneumonia. His presenting symptoms included increased weakness, elevated blood pressure, productive cough, fever and chills. MB was admitted to our medical unit two days prior to Ramadan (the Muslim fasting month). MB was compliant with care and testing and was progressing toward the expected goals.

Suddenly, MB refused all oral medications and all meals and became progressively weaker but could not tell staff what was happening. With the help of an interpreter, staff realized that MB was observing his religion as a devoted Muslim. In accordance with the Islamic tenets, MB would be required to pray 5 times daily, fast for 30 days during Ramadan, and abstain from eating pork. As well, staff learned that male-female physical contact was considered an aberration.

We held an interdisciplinary meeting on how to care for this patient while respecting his religious rights. The attending physician changed MB's medications to the intravenous (IV) route. All female medical team members avoided hugging or handshaking in respect of MB's culture. To meet his psychosocial needs, family visits were encouraged and interpreter services maintained. Within 24 hours of implementing this culturally congruent treatment plan, MB became happier, more compliant and was discharged home within the next two days.

Had a cultural assessment been completed on admission, we would have recognized MB's sudden behavior changes. This situation aligns with Madeleine Leininger's Theory of Culture Care Diversity and Universality, which considers the impact of culture on an individual's health and caring practices. Current evidence shows that practicing nurses have access to a wealth of culturally based research data to carry out optimal, quality care for clients of diverse cultures or subcultures (Alligood, 2018). (RN to BS student)

THE SCIENCE OF PROVIDING PATIENT-CENTERED CARE: THE PICKER INSTITUTE

In 1986, businessman, educator, inventor, and philanthropist Dr. Harvey Picker founded the Boston-based Picker Institute, a not-for-profit organization dedicated to developing a patient-centered approach to health care. Dr. Picker believed that the American health-care system was technologically and scientifically outstanding. Glaringly absent, he felt, was the overall responsiveness to patients' concerns and comfort levels (Frampton & Guastello, 2008).

Over the course of 7 years, Picker and his team interviewed more than 8,000 patients, family members, physicians, and hospital staff about their personal interactions with the health-care system. Findings indicated that patients lacked a trusting relationship with their providers, received insufficient information about their care, and experienced poor communication between themselves and their health-care providers. These themes became the foundation for the Picker Survey, the first-ever patient-centered performance measurement tool. This initiative led to the coining of the term **patient-centered care**. With the development of the first scientifically validated patient-experience survey, patients' interactions with the

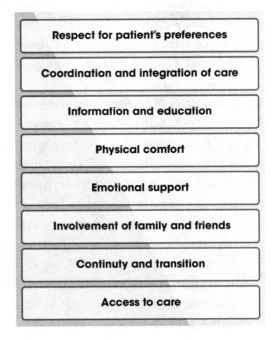

Figure 3.1 Eight Picker Principles of Patient-Centered Care

health-care delivery system were documented, culminating in the **Eight Picker Principles of Patient-Centered Care** (Picker Institute, 2013b).

Despite the history of, and widespread attention to, patient-centered care, meaningful engagement with patients continues to be a challenge. Many organizations are still doing things *to* or *for* patients and their families instead of partnering with them. A patient-centered, health-care structure strengthens relationships among patients, their families, and their providers. With this type of communication, patients should always know where to go and which individuals to approach to have their questions or concerns addressed. Patient engagement should extend to relationships among staff. Ultimately, if staff members are not interacting effectively with one another, or feel unsupported by the administration, the staff-patient relationship will not prosper.

Effective measurement of patient-centered care is daunting. While the Hospital Consumer Assessment of Healthcare Providers and Systems provides nationally standardized comparative information, it does not measure those issues important to patients and families. Qualitative feedback from patients is detailed and valuable, but many health-care organizations struggle with how to use this data effectively to monitor and measure performance. Listening to patients' stories creates the rigor with qualitative metrics that health providers need to improve the patient experience (Picker Institute, 2013a).

OVERVIEW OF PICKER'S EIGHT PRINCIPLES OF PATIENT-CENTERED CARE

1. RESPECT FOR PATIENTS' VALUES, PREFERENCES, AND EXPRESSED NEEDS. All health care providers must involve patients in decision making, acknowledging that they possess distinct values and preferences. Providers need to demonstrate empathy, respect and sensitivity related to patients' cultural values and independence

2. COORDINATION AND INTEGRATION OF CARE. Patients in the focus groups reported feeling vulnerable and helpless during their illness. Collaboration among providers invested in the plan of care can significantly improve the patient experience. Patients recognized that coordination of clinical care, ancillary and support services can impact communication and reduce feelings of vulnerability.

3. INFORMATION AND EDUCATION. Patients interviewed revealed they felt uninformed regarding their conditions, diagnoses and prognoses. By involving patients in discussions about their clinical status, their progress and prognosis, providers can inspire patients' autonomy as well as compliance with treatment.

4. PHYSICAL COMFORT. Patients reported that achieving physical comfort significantly affected their hospital experience. Pain management was linked to the level of assistance needed with activities in the hospital environment and

surroundings (such as patient transfer to x-ray, physical and occupational therapy).

5. *EMOTIONAL SUPPORT AND ALLEVIATION OF FEAR AND ANXIETY.* The impact of illness on patients and their families, coupled with loss of employment and subsequent financial burdens, are major stressors during hospitalization. The continual emotional support and collaboration of the health care provider team with the patient and family can significantly reduce fears related to patient diagnosis, plan of care, treatments and prognosis.

6. *INVOLVEMENT OF FAMILY AND FRIENDS.* Focus group participants recognized family involvement as key in providing patient-centered care. Providing accommodations for family, involving family in decision making and recognizing and supporting the needs of caregivers are all important elements of this principle.

7. *CONTINUITY AND TRANSITION.* Patients reported concerns post discharge regarding self-care. Providers and health care organizations can assist here by ensuring that detailed information regarding home care, (to include medications, physical limitations, home environment barriers, dietary needs, community resources and support services) are in place.

8. *ACCESS TO CARE.* Patients expressed the importance of knowing how to access care when needed. Their health care literacy needs included transportation, physical access to health care organizations/clinics, guidance with the ability to schedule office visits and information on scheduling referral appointments.

NURSING EDUCATION REFORM

IOM Future of Nursing Report

In 2010, IOM published a report with recommendations for nurses on the mission to improve health care in the United States. The goal of the IOM *Future of Nursing* report was as follows:

> *The Future of Nursing: Leading Change, Advancing Health* was to provide a direction for nursing's role in the shift from hospital-based services to a system focused on health promotion in the community. Inspired by the need to include more information in nursing education about the Institute of Medicine (IOM, 2001) reports, The Carnegie Foundation Report (2010) and the National League for Nursing position statement (NLN, 2003), leaders called for nursing education reform on quality health care, with a focus on the five core competencies identified by the IOM for all healthcare professions: 1) patient-centered care, 2) teamwork and collaboration, 3) evidence-based practice, 4) quality improvement, and 5) informatics. (IOM, 2011)

The quality and safety education for nurses (QSEN) model, described by the American Association of Colleges of Nursing (QSEN, 2013), contributed to the competency of safety. QSEN emphasizes competence in maintaining patient safety and delineates the most current trends in nursing practice. Awareness of nursing practice provides the foundation needed to further define and develop care coordination in both academia and in practice (IOM, 2011).

The Robert Wood Johnson Foundation (RWJF) launched a campaign to advance the *Future of Nursing* report's recommendations, creating action coalitions across the United States. A major initiative involved increasing the number of nurses with baccalaureate degrees to 80% in 2020. In 2010, 49% of employed nurses in the United States had BSN degrees compared to 56% in 2017, according to IOM report updates. In California, the percentage of BSN graduates increased from 54% in 2010 to 60% in 2017. Much of that progress can be attributed to the fact that the state's action coalition worked to foster academic partnerships between universities and community colleges (Thew, 2019).

A second IOM *Future of Nursing* goal to improve access to care involved increasing the number of nurse practitioners employed as primary care providers. Many states have removed legal barriers that formerly restricted nurse practitioner practice. In 2016, the Veterans Administration agreed to allow nurse practitioners, clinical nurse specialists, and nurse-midwives to practice without the supervision of a physician, regardless of the practice restrictions in the state where the facility is located (U.S. Department of Veteran Affairs, 2016).

A further objective highlighted in the report concerned the need to increase diversity in the nursing workforce. The rationale for this recommendation was to enable a better understanding of factors affecting overall patient health (IOM, 2011). In 2017, 30% of all graduates were minority nursing students, an increase of 7% in 2010. This growth is inadequate when considering that Hispanics and Latinos, who represent nearly 20% of the U.S. population, comprise less than 10% of the nursing workforce.

Dr. Karren Kowalski, president and CEO of the Colorado Center for Nursing Excellence, was concerned about the lack of diversity in her state's nursing workforce. With a RWJF research grant, Kowalski and colleagues discovered that minority nursing students were leaving academia. Securing Human Resources and Services Administration funding, the team created a program for nurses to become mentors to nursing students. With a 90% graduation rate annually, the outcomes demonstrate that the program has been successful (Kowalski, 2012; Kowalski, 2015).

An additional recommendation from the RWJF and the IOM (2011) urged nurses to collaborate with health-care professionals in reshaping the country's health-care system. RWJF partnered with AARP (American Association of Retired Persons) to establish the *Campaign for Action*, a program created to instill nursing knowledge and experience into community organizations, with the ultimate goal of helping individuals to lead longer, healthier lives. To increase the number of nurses on boards, the *Campaign for Action* helped fund the *Nurses on Boards Coalition*, which matches nurses with boards (such as health facilities, schools, businesses, city planning) that align with their areas of interest and expertise. The goal of the *Nurses on Boards Coalition* was to increase that number to 10,000 by 2020 (Altman et al., 2016).

NURSING THEORIES RELATED TO PATIENT-CENTERED CARE

Leininger's theory of culture care diversity and universality (Alligood, 2018) considers the effect of culture on an individual's health and caring practices. The definition of patient-centered care, according to the IOM (2011), includes addressing cultural aspects and health-care disparities as treatment goals congruent with cultural values, beliefs, and practices. Leininger's sunrise model (Melo, 2013) incorporates three cultural care concepts (1) maintenance/preservation, (2) negotiation/accommodation, and (3) restructuring/repatterning) in the provision of patient-centered care.

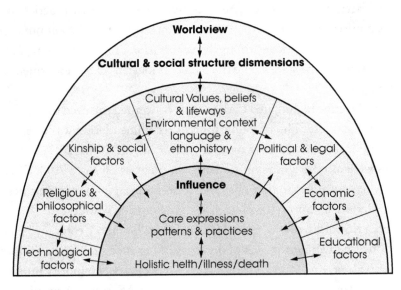

Figure 3.2 Sunshine Model

Cultural preservation refers to nursing support of individual cultural practices, such as employing acupressure for anxiety or pain prior to medical interventions. Correspondingly, cultural negotiation refers to the support provided to patients and families in regard to cultural activities that do not pose threats to patients or other individuals in the health-care setting. Finally, cultural restructuring involves nurses' efforts to deliver patient-centered care by helping patients modify or change their cultural activities. Cultural restructuring is recommended when cultural practices risk harming patients and others in the surrounding environment. These concepts can inform nurses in ways of achieving optimal patient-centered care goals (Melo, 2013).

Orem's self-care theory incorporates nursing's empowerment of patients to become full participants in their own care (Alligood, 2018). Consisting of those activities performed independently by an individual to promote and maintain personal well-being, self-care is identified by the IOM (2011) as an essential component of patient-centered care. The nurse meets the self-care needs of patients by guiding, teaching, supporting, or providing settings conducive to promoting the patient's abilities. Self-care implies that a partnership between the patient and the professional is established where problems are identified, and appropriate interventions are determined. Patient participation is crucial for the development of the plan of care itself to foster independence (Orem, 1995).

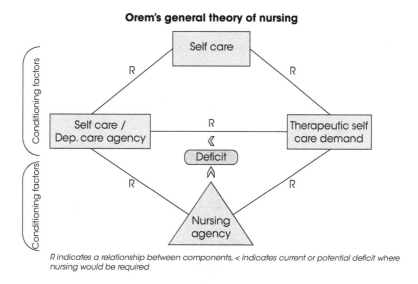

Figure 3.3 Orem's Model

To implement patient-centered care, Orem (1995) proposed three "moments." Initially, the nurse meets the individual with health-care needs. This contact has to be established, legitimized, and adequate according to the evidence required by nursing. The nurse identifies the requirements, systems, and new self-care needs, as well as diagnosis and nursing prescriptions. In the second step, the nurse creates a system to address ways to care for the patient, with input supplied by family members or caregivers. The third step involves preparing the patient, family, or person responsible for the self-care to become independent of the nurse's actions. An agreement is established with the patient and includes discussion about possible barriers that might interfere during this new adjustment (Orem, 1995).

Peplau's interpersonal relations theory (Peplau, 1997) stresses the importance of therapeutic communication in initiating the nurse-patient relationship. Peplau's theory encompasses seven nursing roles: (1) stranger, (2) resource, (3) teacher, (4) counselor, (5) surrogate, (6) active leader, and (7) technical expert (Peplau, 1992). The theory is described as an interpersonal therapeutic process occurring as nurses establish relationships with those needing health services. Peplau theorized that nurse-patient relationships move through three phases: (1) orientation, (2) working, and (3) termination.

During the orientation phase, hospitalized patients recognize that they need help as they attempt to cope with their current experience. Concurrently, nurses meet patients and identify their unique needs and priorities (Peplau, 1997). Among the many roles that nurses assume in their interactions with patients, the first role during the orientation phase is that of stranger. Initially, nurses are expected to greet all patients with respect and positive interest (Peplau, 1952).

The working phase accounts for the majority of nurses' time with patients. Nurses make assessments about patients when contributing to an interdisciplinary plan of care. During the working phase, nurses' roles become more familiar to patients. They begin to accept nurses as health educators, resource persons, counselors, and care providers. Nurses practice "nondirective listening" to facilitate patients' increased awareness of their feelings regarding their changing health (Peplau, 1952).

The final phase is termination, where discharge planning takes place (Peplau, 1992). The success of the termination phase is dependent on how well patients and nurses navigate the orientation and working phases. A major part of the termination phase occurs when nurses teach patients about symptom management and recovery at home.

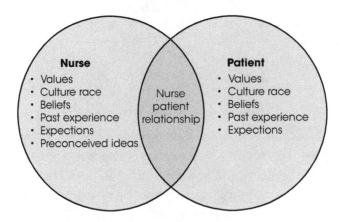

Figure 3.4 Peplau Model

Peplau emphasized that careful, active listening is extremely important. She reported that the nurse's behavior signals a pattern of receptivity and interest in the patient's concerns, either of which can succeed or fail in this respect. Peplau asserted that the center of scientific research in nursing should be patients, their needs, and their perceptions about the care they received from nurses (Peplau, 1992).

Watson's caring theory maintains that care is patient centered, highlights caring as an important tenet, and describes how nurses incorporate caring in practice (Watson, 2011). Caring consists of 10 "carative" causes. Watson uses the term "carative" rather than "curative" to distinguish between nursing and medicine. Curative factors aim at curing the patient of disease, whereas carative factors aim at the caring process that helps the person attain or maintain health (Watson, 2008).

Actions by nurses in daily practice involve patients on every level: establishing a caring relationship, using a holistic approach, displaying unconditional acceptance and positive regard, and promoting health through knowledge and interventions. Based on the premise that nurses are healers through kindness and through meeting the holistic needs of patients, caring theory encourages nurses to be "authentically present" for patients. Also, the theory discusses the need for nurses to search their own beliefs and care for their own emotional and spiritual needs (Watson, 2006).

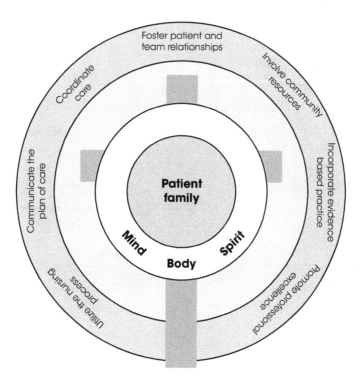

Figure 3.5 Watson Model

The core of nursing is caring for others and for oneself. Nurses must be able to establish personal contact, demonstrate therapeutic communication, and sustain positive interpersonal relationships with patients. Interventions should reflect professionalism and care for individual problems, not daily tasks to be accomplished. As well, caring is important for the well-being of staff working with patients. The environment and culture in health-care institutions have a significant impact on nurses' perceptions of carative factors.

The promotion of a supportive, protective, holistic patient care setting empowers nurses to engage in caring partnerships with patients. Emphasis on caring theories is essential from the start of one's nursing education, as part of lifelong learning in the profession. In this way, a strong core of knowledge related to caring theories and evidence-based practice can exist.

PERSON-CENTERED CARE: THEORY IN PRACTICE

Person-centered care (Rogers, 1959) encompasses knowledge of the individual as a whole person. The process often involves the input of family members to assist patients in assessing their own needs and planning their own care. Contrary to this method is a task-focused approach, where Maslow's hierarchy of needs prioritizes physical tasks over holistic care (Rollin, 2011). While person-centered care should consistently guide nursing practice, it can sometimes be forgotten during the daily delivery of patient care in a hectic and demanding health-care setting.

Rogers (1959) believed individuals learn throughout their lives and are capable of achieving personal growth through unconditional positive regard within trusting, genuine, and open relationships. Self-actualization leads to self-confidence and self-esteem, leading to new feelings, new experiences, and new knowledge. Conversely, feelings of insecurity compromise physical and mental health, limiting nurses' ability to fully care for patients.

In person-centered care (Durant et al., 2015), caring is central to nursing practice, and nurses' relationships with

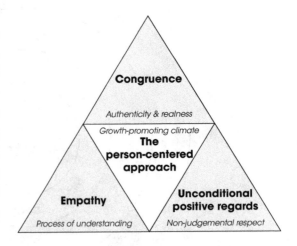

Figure 3.6 Rogers Person Centered Care Model

the person (patient) are fundamental to that individual's experiences of care. The patient role is one of partnership rather than passivity. The move from a dependent receiver of care to an empowered partner in care requires a trusting relationship. In an environment of caring, nurses advocate for and support patients' needs to express their fears, which ultimately promotes self-caring behavior. The humanistic concepts supporting person-centered care incorporate respect for individuals and their rights to self-determination, mutual esteem, and empathy (McCormack et al., 2011).

PATIENT-CENTERED CARE: IMPLICATIONS FOR NURSING PRACTICE

Chapman (2017) advised that focusing on nursing tasks and "nurse knows best" (p.9) attitudes convey total apathy for and disinterest in the individual patient. Instead, nurses are encouraged to take their lead from patients during interactions regarding their interests, fears, and needs. Viewing patients' situations through their own eyes and acknowledging their understanding of the care to be delivered through careful explanation and evaluation of feedback fosters a foundation of trust between patient and caregiver. When initiated early on in the nurse-patient relationship, these actions ultimately empower patients to make informed decisions and become active participants in their care.

Durant et al. (2015) reported on the 2010 efforts of California's Kaiser Permanente (KP) leaders and providers to integrate caring science beliefs into their organization. Based on Jean Watson's theory (Watson, 2006; Watson, 2011), caring science serves as an essential practice guide for nursing professionals. In this study, caregivers at KP endeavored to balance the art and science of clinical judgment by addressing the holistic needs of patients and involving them in decisions that fostered their well-being. Durant et al. (2015) sought to disseminate evidence on how a professional practice framework, such as caring science (Watson, 2008), could transform the caring-healing practice, the environment, and the culture across a large organizational hospital system. Also, the authors endeavored to provide evidence on how integration of caring science across administrative, operational, and clinical areas can lead to significant quality health outcomes for patients.

Outcomes from the study (Durant et al., 2015) demonstrated that the caring science practice model, implemented throughout a large, 21-center, health-care organization, inspired health-care workers and providers by reminding them of the purpose and value of their work. Staff recognized and were transformed by the connection between their own values and the strategic initiatives that guided practice within their hospital organization. The authors believe that these encouraging study findings should drive further research related to caring science's ability to "transform the ethic of caring-healing practice, environment, and culture" (Durant et al., 2015, p. 141).

FOSTERING PATIENT PARTICIPATION IN DECISION MAKING

Working in the health-care field requires sound communication skills. Effectively communicating with patients, families, and other health-care providers is the foundation for a therapeutic, positive patient experience. Patients' care experiences are greatly influenced by what is communicated and observed through their subjective and objective feedback. As health-care providers, nurses affect and are affected by these patient interactions.

Whether it is advocating for or establishing rapport with patients and families or communicating with other members of the interprofessional team, the nurse's ability to communicate effectively is constantly challenged. Thinking before acting on first impressions is key. Also, building positive communication and rapport at the outset has been linked to more favorable patient care ratings (Kourkouta & Papathanasiou, 2014).

Rubenfeld and Scheffer (2014) offer several recommendations for nurses and other health-care providers when communicating with patients about the need to participate in formulating their plan of care. Nurses must be aware of their own body language, as well as the body language of their patients, and what this language conveys. The nurse entering the patient's room to find the individual lying in a fetal position, facing the wall, could evoke a myriad of signals: sleep, pain, depression, or fear. It is important for the nurse to avoid assumptions and to validate what the patient is truly experiencing in the moment.

To foster participation and compliance during an initial meeting with patients, Rubenfeld and Scheffer (2014) recommended asking them how they wish to be addressed. This action conveys respect and interest in patients as individuals. A statement such as, "This is Mr. S, but he prefers to be called Pete," rather than "the heart patient in Room 325," can make an appreciable difference in the way patients accept treatments and care.

Maintain presence by entering the patient's room. Avoid talking to patients from the doorway. Sitting down beside a patient puts you at eye level and conveys interest, empathy, and an investment in their situation. This action typically elicits subjective assessment data, such as determining patients' knowledge of why they are hospitalized. Fostering further communication through open-ended questions, which typically stimulate much more than a "yes" or "no" answer) alerts the nurse to particular areas of concern and prioritizes interventions. Using collaborative language ("what do you think about …?") conveys the message that the nurse is interested in planning care of the patient with the patient. Also, this approach to collaborative care promotes awareness of individual patient needs, such as cultural norms, dietary concerns, spiritual practices, and personal space issues.

Nurses are resourceful, creative, and critical thinkers, but the challenge to meet patients' needs in the current health-care climate is formidable. Patient hospital stays are short-term. Staffing ratios are inadequate. There is no "one size fits all" approach to care or to the ethical dilemmas that nurses face daily in the workplace. Adding the tools of early assessment, maintaining presence, body language awareness, and collaborative communication can fully complement those practice skills already in place in the delivery of safe, professional, and compassionate patient care.

TRANSPARENCY IN COMMUNICATION

A lack of transparency results in distrust and a deep sense of insecurity.

—*Dalai Lama*

Key to building trust, transparency in communication is a valuable skill. People who communicate honestly, openly, and authentically are more credible, more often heard, and considered more trustworthy. Research indicates that great leaders are open communicators and good listeners.

Their messages are clear, straightforward, and consistent. Transparent communication is essential to managing and leading others successfully, as clear and honest communication builds trust. Without trust, transparent relationships cannot grow (Jahromi et al., 2016; Kourkouta & Papathanasiou, 2014).

During staff meetings, transparency in communication can be challenging for all parties, particularly when the information is both difficult to deliver and to hear. As a meeting facilitator, supervisor, or manager, possessing conflict resolution skills is essential. Preparing in advance by obtaining current, accurate information from all parties involved helps to maintain a calm, neutral environment, one that is private and secure. Introducing ground rules, such as "each person will speak, one at a time" and paraphrasing after each person speaks, clarifies what is being said and corrects any misperceptions. The goal for all parties involved is to leave the meeting with a mutually agreed upon, concrete plan to resolve the conflict.

Jahromi et al. (2016) recommended that leaders share with staff their own fears during difficult times regarding the unknown. This action shows vulnerability as a leader, encourages staff feedback, respects staff members' opinions, and demonstrates the leader's ability to empathize with staff members' own fears. Also, clarifying information during a crisis and promising to update staff members as soon as new information is known can create an atmosphere of sincerity, honesty, and respect (Jahromi et al., 2016; Kourkouta & Papathanasiou, 2014).

SOCIAL DETERMINANTS OF HEALTH

Never doubt that a small group of thoughtful, committed, citizens can change the world. Indeed, it is the only thing that ever has.

– *Margaret Mead*

Despite technological and biological advances in health care, less progress has been made in addressing social determinants of health (SDH). The World Health Organization defines SDH as those conditions into which people are born, grow, live, work, and age, and those systems influencing the conditions of daily life (WHO, 2018). SDH include such factors as socioeconomic status, environment (including air and water quality), food insecurity and food safety, education, employment, social networks, homelessness, and racism (Thornton & Persaud, 2018).

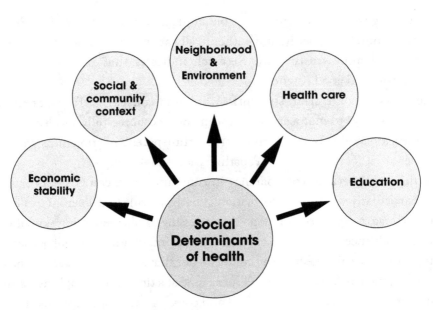

Figure 3.7 Social Determinants of Health

In 2016, the Dana-Farber/Boston Children's Cancer and Blood Disorders Center reported that children with acute lymphoblastic leukemia who are poor are more likely to suffer earlier relapses (Bona et al., 2016). Although more study is needed to understand the connection between SDH and health outcomes, poor families' lack of resources may be one explanation. Poverty and homelessness can both contribute to and result from health problems. With exposure to contagious conditions, homelessness can lead to further illness. Stress and violence also have a significant influence on both physical and mental health (Bona et al., 2016).

A goal of the Healthy People 2020 initiative is to construct environments that will foster health.

Also, the Code of Ethics for Nurses includes principles of social justice and emphasizes the need to integrate social concerns into nursing and health policy. Beginning in entry level nursing education curriculum and integrated in all health-care settings during patient assessment and care, student nurses should be taught, and practicing nurses should be encouraged, to adopt the role of change agent in advocating for improvements in SDH. Through grassroots efforts of participation and volunteerism in shelters, food pantries, clinics, and other local community agencies, change can take place. Offering skills and collaborating with representatives of social work, public health, city planning, police, and fire fighters, nurses can raise awareness of resources, space, people, equipment, and policies that are either available or that need to be enabled to address the SDH in one's community (Thornton & Persaud, 2018).

HEALTHY PEOPLE 2020

Healthy People 2020, a 10-year national agenda, is a tool to identify health priorities and improve the nation's health by shifting the focus from treating diseases to preventing them. The Healthy People initiative was established in 1980 with the release of "Healthy People 1990." Members of the U.S. Department of Health and Human Services (2020), together with public health and other government officials, collaborated to create a framework to address and prioritize major health issues in the United States (Office of Disease Prevention and Health Promotion, 2018).

The Healthy People 2020 framework is composed of goals to track progress in areas of health, ranging from heart disease and stroke to cancer, nutrition, immunizations, and oral health. The campaign's purpose is to identify and reduce health disparities by focusing on those factors that affect an individual's health status, such as education, housing, transportation, and poverty. Goals involve achieving the following: longer high-quality lives free of preventable disease, disability, injury, and premature death; health equity by improving the health of all groups; social and physical environments that promote good health for all; and healthy development and behaviors across all life stages.

PROVIDING CULTURALLY SENSITIVE CARE

Nurses work in a wide variety of settings, including hospitals, schools, day care, correctional facilities and community health. Employment in such diverse settings, in a growing global society, suggests that nurses are likely to care for individuals from many different cultural backgrounds and beliefs. Regardless of an individual's cultural beliefs and practices, nurses have the responsibility to provide culturally sensitive, ethical care to all patients (Giger, 2016).

Autonomy is the ethical principle of respecting the rights of patients to make their own decisions, even if those decisions conflict with the values of the nurse. For the nurse, a significant part of supporting this autonomy is in developing awareness of the patient's culture. However, while culture can be defined as a group's beliefs, it cannot be assumed that patients embrace certain cultural traditions because they identify with a certain eth-nicity or religion. It is critical, however, that nurses understand the patient's own culture, as culture includes how patients perceive health and illness. Including patients in the plan of care assures patients' autonomy and ensures that cultural beliefs will be integrated into that care (Gouvere & Gouvere, 2016; Ong-Flaherty, 2015).

More than ever, as the population continues to grow, cultural diversity and awareness have become an integral part of health care. As providers, nurses care for many vulnera-ble, diverse populations and work with diverse staff (Bhatt & Bathia, 2018). Culture and life experiences shape both patients' and nurses' worldviews about health, illness, and health care.

Strategies to facilitate communication, increase understanding, and reduce stress when providing culturally congruent care include providers' self-education and empow-erment regarding cultural awareness and sensitivity, teaching by demonstration, giving simple explanations, and demonstrating empathy. When providers attend to culturally specific meaning in all interactions with patients, they create and support trusting rela-tionships. Hopefully, this mindset will contribute to reducing racial and ethnic disparities in health-care services and lead to positive health outcomes for all patient populations (Marion et al, 2016.

CHAPTER SUMMARY

The IOM core competency of patient-centered care was the overarching concept guid-ing the content of Chapter 3. With an overview of the origin of patient-centered care and its related principles, readers examined current challenges and opportunities in health care. Discussions in the chapter included IOM competencies, Healthy People 2020 goals, SDH, and cultural awareness and sensitivity. These are key elements in planning and providing holistic, culturally congruent, professional, and safe care for all patient populations. As lifelong learners and critical thinkers, nurses are readily equipped to integrate this evidence into a theory-based practice.

FOOD FOR THOUGHT: CRITICAL THINKING QUESTIONS

1. Describe the origin and significance of "patient-centered care" principles.
2. Identify strategies to fulfill the IOM *Future of Nursing* patient-centered care competencies.
3. Compare the caring theories of nurses (Leininger, Orem, Peplau, and Watson) as they relate to the concept of patient-centered care.

4. Discuss communication techniques to foster patient participation in and compliance with creating an individualized plan of care.
5. Review the Healthy People 2020 national initiative recommendations for addressing SDH.
6. Recognize the relationship between culture and diversity and current health-care delivery in the United States.

SCENARIO: CULTURALLY SENSITIVE CARE

Margaret is a registered nurse at a local family health clinic. The clinic's client population consists of native-born, low-income families, as well as a large immigrant population. Margaret, white and native-born, has been working with Joy, an immigrant from Cambodia who speaks English proficiently, and Jessica, her 7-month-old. Mother and baby are here at the clinic today for well child visit and scheduled immunizations. Margaret observes a happy baby, with growth and developmental indicators normal for her age. As she continues with the assessment, Margaret notes several red skin eruptions on the baby's buttocks and thighs. When asked about the marks, Joy looks at the floor and states she has not noticed them before.

1. What questions come to mind about the above scenario?
2. How should the nurse proceed?
3. What information would help clarify the issues raised?

NURSING JOURNAL: REFLECT ON YOUR PRACTICE WHILE HONING YOUR WRITING SKILLS

The "Culture" of Nursing

Today's nursing workforce consists of staff and nursing leaders from different generational cohorts. Generational diversity, including workforce differences in attitudes, beliefs, work habits, and expectations, has proven challenging for nurses and nursing administrations. Describe the "culture" of the health organization where you practice. Give examples of both strengths and challenges in this setting as it relates to the nursing culture of caring for patients. What are your recommendations to enhance personal and professional growth regarding encouraging the multigenerational workforce to thrive and to meet future health-care challenges? Please cite literature and use examples from your practice to support your response.

CHAPTER 3 REFERENCES

Alligood, M. (2018). *Nursing theorists and their work* (9th ed.). Elsevier.

Altman S., Butler, A. & Shern, L. (Eds.). (2016). *Assessing progress on implementing the recommendations of the institute of medicine report. The Future of Nursing: Leading Change, Advancing Health.* National Academies Press. https://www.ncbi.nlm.nih.gov/books/NBK350168/

Bhatt, J., & Bathia, P. (2018) Ensuring access to quality health care in vulnerable communities. *Academic Medicine, 93*(9), 1271–1275. https://doi.org/10.1097/ACM.0000000000002254

Bona, K., Blonquist, T., Neuberg, D., Silverman, L. B., & Wolfe, J. (2016). Impact of socioeconomic status on timing of relapse and overall survival for children treated on Dana-Farber Cancer Institute ALL consortium protocols (2000–2010). *Pediatric Blood and Cancer, 63*(6), 1012–1018.

Chapman, H. (2017). Nursing theories 1: Person-centered care. *Nursing Times, 113*(10), 59.

Durant, A., McDermott, S., Kinney, G.,Triner, T., & Perm, J. (2015). Caring science: Transforming the ethic of caring-healing practice, environment, and culture within an integrated care delivery system. *Nursing Research and Practice, 19*(4), e136-e142. http://dx.doi.org/10.7812/TPP/15-042

Frampton, S., & Guastello, S. (2008). Honoring the life of a pioneer in patient-centered care: Harvey Picker. *The Patient: Patient-Centered Outcomes Research, 1*(2). https://doi.org/10.2165/01312067-200801020-00001

Giger, J. (2016). *Transcultural nursing: Assessment and intervention.* Elsevier Health Sciences.

Govere, L. & Govere, E. (2016). How effective is cultural competence training of healthcare providers on improving patient satisfaction of minority groups? A systematic review of literature. *Worldviews on Evidence-Based Nursing, 13*(6), 402–410.

Institute of Medicine (IOM). (2001). *Crossing the quality chasm: A new health system for the 21st century.* National Academy Press.

Institute of Medicine (IOM). (2011). *The future of nursing: Leading change, advancing health.* National Academies Press. https://www.ncbi.nlm.nih.gov/books/NBK209885/

Jahromi, V., Tabatabase, S., Abdar, Z., & Raiabi, M. (2016). Active listening: The key of successful communication in hospital managers. *Electronic Physician, 8*(3), 2123–2128. https://doi.org/10.19082/2123 PMCID: PMC4844478

Kourkouta, L., & Papathanasiou, I. (2014). Communication in nursing practice. *Materia Socio-Medica, 26*(1), 65–67. https://doi.org/10.5455/msm.2014.26.65-67 PMCID: PMC3990376

Kowalski, K. (2012). Recommendations of the future of nursing report. *Journal of Continuing Education in Nursing, 43*(2), 57–58. https://doi.org/10.3928/00220124-20120125-04

Kowalski K. (2015). Nurses on boards. *Journal of Continuing Education in Nursing, 46*(11), 489–491. https://doi.org/10.3928/00220124-20151020-14

Marion, L., Douglas, M., Lavin, M., Barr, N., Gazaway, S., Thomas, L., & Bickford, C. (2016). Implementing the new ANA standard 8: Culturally congruent practice" *OJIN: The Online Journal of Issues in Nursing, 22*(1).

McCormack, B., Dewing, J., & McCance, T. (2011). Developing person-centered care: Addressing contextual challenges through practice development. *Online Journal of Issues in Nursing, 16*(2), 3.

Melo, L. P. D. (2013). The sunrise model: A contribution to the teaching of nursing consultation in collective health. *American Journal of Nursing Research, 1*(1), 20–23.

Office of Disease Prevention and Health Promotion. (2018). Maternal, infant, and child health. In U.S. Department of Health and Human Services (Ed.)., *Healthy people 2020* **(pp. 1–7).** https://www.healthypeople.gov/2020/topics-objectives/topic/maternal-infant-and-child-health/objectives

Ong-Flaherty, C. (2015). Critical cultural awareness and diversity in nursing: A minority perspective. *Nurse Leader, 13*(5), 58–62. http://dx.doi.org/10.1016/j.mnl.2015.03.012

Orem, D. E. (1995). *Nursing: Concepts of practice* (5th ed.). Mosby.

Peplau H. E. (1952). *Interpersonal relations in nursing.* Putnam.

Peplau H. E. (1992) Interpersonal relations: A theoretical framework for application in nursing practice. *Nursing Science Quarterly, 5,* 13–18.

Peplau, H. E. (1997). Peplau's theory of interpersonal relations. *Nursing Science Quarterly, 10*(4), 162–167. https://doi.org/10.1177/089431849701000407

Picker Institute. (2013a). *Patient-centered care: The road ahead.* https://ipfcc.org/resources/Patient-Centered-Care-The-Road-Ahead.pdf

Picker Institute. (2013b). *Picker principles of patient centered care.* http://www.pickereurope.org/about-us/principles-of-patient-centred-care/

Quality and Safety Education for Nurses (QSEN). (2013). *Project overview: The evolution of the quality and safety education for nurses' initiative.* http://qsen.org/about-qsen/project-overview/

Rogers, C. (1959) A theory of therapy, personality and interpersonal relationships as developed in the client centered framework. In S. Koch (Ed.), *Psychology: A study of a science (pp. 207–213; 223–244).* McGraw Hill.

Rollin, H. (2011). Practical care: How to improve care plans. *Nursing and Residential Care, 13,* 541–543.

Rubenfeld, M., & Scheffer, B. (2014) *Critical thinking tactics for nurses.* Jones and Bartlett.

Thew, J. (2019, March 15). *The future of nursing report: Where are we now? Health Leaders.* Retrieved February 26, 2020, from https://www.healthleadersmedia.com/nursing/future-nursing-report-where-are-we-now

Thornton, M., & Persaud, S. (2018). Preparing today's nurses: Social determinants of health and nursing education" *OJIN: The Online Journal of Issues in Nursing, 23* (3), 1–12. https://doi.org/10.3912/OJIN.Vol23No03Man05

U.S. Department of Health and Human Services. (2020). *Healthy people 2020.* https://www.healthypeople.gov/2020/topics-objectives/topic/maternal-infant-and-child-health/objectives

U.S. Department of Veteran Affairs (2016). *VA grants full practice authority to advanced practice registered nurses.* https://www.va.gov/opa/pressrel/includes/viewPDF.cfm?id=2847

Watson, J. (2006). Caring theory as an ethical guide to administrative and clinical practices. *Nursing Administration Quarterly, 30*(1), 48–55. http://dx.doi. org/10.1097/00006216-200601000-00008.

Watson, J. (2008). *Nursing: The philosophy and science of caring* (rev. ed.). University Press of Colorado.

Watson, J. (2011). *Caring science: a theory of nursing* (2nd ed.). Jones & Bartlett.

World Health Organization (WHO). (2018). *Closing the gap in a generation: Health equity through action on the social determinants of health. Commission on Social Determinants of Health.* http://www.who.int/social_determinants/en

ADDITIONAL RESOURCES

https://www.cms.gov/Medicare/Quality-Initiatives-Patient-Assessment

https://www.cms.gov/Medicare/Quality-Initiatives-Patient-Assessment-Instruments/HospitalQualityInits

CREDITS

Fig. 3.1: Source: https://www.oneviewhealthcare.com/blog/the-eight-principles-of-patient-centered-care/.

Fig. 3.2: Adapted from Source: http://pubs.sciepub.com/ajnr/1/1/3/.

Fig. 3.3: Adapted from Source: https://www.researchgate.net/figure/Conceptual-model-Orem-s-theory-of-self-care-nursing-R-relationship-deR-cit_fig1_13503185.

Fig. 3.4: Source: https://rnspeak.com/hildegard-peplau-nursing-theory/.

Fig. 3.5: Source: https://www.slideshare.net/sinsu12/jean-watson-theory-of-human-care.

Fig. 3.6: Adapted from Source: https://counsellingtutor.com/counselling-approaches/person-centred-approach-to-counselling/carl-rogers-core-conditions/.

Fig. 3.7: Adapted from Source: https://health.gov/healthypeople/objectives-and-data/social-determinants-health.

Work in Interprofessional Teams

CHAPTER INTRODUCTION

In Chapter 4, the reader will examine strategies that empower nurses as agents of change. Discussion centers on communication and interprofessional collaboration. Relevant IOM competencies and ANA standards, shared/professional governance models of communication handoff tools, and the challenges of implementing collaborative care are explored. The intent of this chapter is to assist the nurse/reader with recognizing, appreciating, and employing those strategies for optimizing quality patient care delivery as a valued member of the interprofessional team.

KEY TERMS: MAKING CONNECTIONS

- Communication
- Handoff tools: SBAR, I-PASS, BSR
- Interprofessional practice and education
- King's theory of goal attainment
- Nursing process
- Shared/professional governance

LEARNING OBJECTIVES/OUTCOMES
At the end of this chapter, students will accomplish the following:

- Examine the IOM's competency of working in interprofessional teams.
- Recognize the effect of communication gaps related to adverse events.
- Identify factors that impact nursing leadership and management.
- Describe the concept of shared/professional governance
- Compare handoff communication tools: SBAR, I-PASS, BSR
- Examine the interpersonal systems of action, reaction, interaction, and trans-action in King's theory of goal attainment and their relationship to the nursing process

> The secret of change is to focus all of your energy not on fighting the old but on building the new.
>
> —*Socrates*

> Mutual respect and a true sharing of both power and control are essential elements of collaboration
>
> —*Virginia Henderson*

A NURSE'S PERSPECTIVE

I had cared for a terminally ill cancer patient who was expecting to go home on hospice. When I came into work that next evening, the day team was discharging this patient. As I was getting the report, a code green (a medical emergency dealing with anyone who is not a patient) was called. The nurse who had accompanied this patient for discharge ran up to our unit, saying that the patient was in respiratory distress (it was later determined that she had experienced a stroke). I immediately paged the nurse supervisor and gestured for my charge nurse to help me, because I knew time might not be on our side. I felt that it was best for the patient to just come right back up to the same room on the same floor and have the same nurse, instead of going through the emergency department (ED) process all over again, to be admitted. The patient had made it clear already she did not want any life-saving measures done. Being placed in a crowded ED, not knowing what might happen, just did not seem ideal for this patient. I was concerned that the patient would pass and the family would have to deal with it in a clustered environment. However, my idea would challenge certain hospital processes and protocols. I quickly explained my position to the nurse supervisor and charge nurse, who both listened attentively and agreed. The nurse supervisor intervened, the patient was brought back to the same room and I was assigned as the nurse. The patient's doctor arrived on the unit; it was determined that the patient would not survive through the night, and she was placed on comfort measures. The family expressed thanks that I would be the nurse again for their loved one. She passed away that night, surrounded by family. As sad as it was, everyone still had a sense of peace and comfort. Although the situation challenged protocols, our team's collaborative decisions were based on the best interests of this patient and her family. (RN to BS student)

THE IOM REPORT AND INTERPROFESSIONAL COLLABORATION

Despite being rated highly by the public for ethical standards and honesty and being considered one of the most trusted sources of health information, nurses often are excluded from decision making and instead delegated to carry out the directives of others (IOM, 2011). *The Future of Nursing* cites that nurses are often the best sources of knowledge and awareness of patients, families, and communities, but they are hesitant to articulate their concerns. The IOM report urged health-care organizations, nursing faculty, and nursing associations to educate, support, and encourage nurses to lead and manage interprofessional collaboration efforts.

The Future of Nursing recommends an increase in opportunities for nurses to collaborate with physicians and other members of the health-care team (IOM, 2011). The report challenges organizations, such as the Center for Medicare & Medicaid Innovation, to support the development of models of care that are headed by nurse leaders. Also, health-care organizations must support nurses to lead the way in pioneering creative, patient-centered care models (IOM, 2011).

INTERPROFESSIONAL PRACTICE AND EDUCATION

According to Nester (2016), the term **interprofessional practice and education** (IPE), rather than multidisciplinary or interdisciplinary care, is a more contemporary term. Nester believed IPE describes those individuals from two or more professions who, rather than working independently of one another, collaborate to learn about each other with the ultimate goal of improving health outcomes. Mutual respect among the professions is critical to help build relationships, interconnections, and interdependencies to address complex problems, such as health-care services. To succeed in today's health-care environment, interprofessional teams are essential.

In a health-care setting, whether long-term care facility, inpatient acute care, or community agency, patients interact with providers from many health disciplines. It is logical, then, that those health-care professionals will be communicating with each other in a productive way to streamline care and maximize benefits to the patient. Trusting this **communication** to develop gradually, however, is not enough to guarantee that every aspect of patient-centered care is accomplished.

In Standard 9, the ANA speaks to the importance of communication (American Nurses Association, 2015a, 2015b). Within this standard, two components are cited by Rossler et al. (2017): assessing one's own communication skills and maintaining effective communication with interprofessional team members (ANA, 2015). In their study, the authors created a collaborative opportunity for students across multiple health disciplines to examine the practice of team-based care (Rossler et al., 2017).

Rossler et al. (2017) believed that coordination by faculty from different departments was essential to the program's success. Together nursing, physical therapy, public health, health administration, speech and language pathology, and respiratory therapy faculty developed the curriculum and simulation experiences, integrating the work into preexisting courses for each degree track (Rossler et al., 2017). The intent was to simulate realistic, collaborative problem solving in the delivery of health care.

The multidisciplinary, collaborative program incorporated a pre-and postevaluation. Surveys were based on each student's self-assessment of both competence and confidence as a participating member of an interprofessional health-care team (Rossler et al., 2017). It was noted in the postassessment survey that students from every department except respiratory therapy showed a statistically significant improvement in their perceived ability, value, and comfort level in working with others (Rossler et al., 2017).

Prior to completing the post-self-assessment on meeting interprofessional teamwork competencies, students and faculty met for a debriefing of the program. The collaborative sharing of ideas raised important perspectives from students across disciplines. Participants disclosed that, prior to the program, their understanding of what other health professionals contributed was minimal (Rossler et al., 2017). Feedback confirmed that in the delivery of effective, patient-centered care, all disciplines need to coordinate, collaborate, and learn from one another. Also, students revealed that working in teams is sometimes difficult but that the benefit to the patient is evident (Rossler et al., 2017).

Overall, the findings were promising. Rossler et al. (2017) believe that the study could be replicated in various universities. Students reported that the program was valuable in the sense that it will be remembered as they continue on in their education. Also, the experience will most likely be recalled as an important aspect of professional practice as students graduate and enter professional practice. Future studies should ensure that all members of the health-care workforce are able to participate in such an immersive experience.

THE INTERPROFESSIONAL TEAM

One member of a health-care team cannot provide all of the clinical and educational services that patients need in today's model of care. Interprofessional teams include individuals, such as physicians/physician assistants, nurses, physical and occupational therapists, nutritionists, pharmacists, social services, mental health workers, community health workers, and informatics specialists.

Adding these individuals to advisory boards, where they are contributing on a larger scale to the care of patients and communities, is vital to communication and strategies for best practices. This teamwork and sharing of values help to break down walls and change fragmentation of care to integration of care. Ultimately, interprofessional teams that leverage information, experience, technology, and a culture of teamwork provide continuity of current, informed quality care for patients and their families (Arena & Lavie, 2015).

INTERPROFESSIONAL HEALTH-CARE CHALLENGES

Interprofessional care teams that are a part of health-care organizations face potential obstacles in their work. In addition, SDHs can create major barriers for team members who are trying to meet the needs of the diverse populations of their patients. A patient in chronic respiratory failure who cannot afford an air conditioner, or a homeless new mother of a premature newborn, are examples of acute, stressful, and challenging situations for the team and the organization.

As reported by administrators, **communication** among team members is their toughest daily challenge. This is particularly evident when teams are caring for the complex needs of patients, compounded by the complexity of having multiple providers for their care. Coordinating communication and updating information on electronic health records (EHR) can also be very demanding and time-consuming, especially when health-care providers are under pressure to meet patient and organizational goals and deadlines for reimbursement (Cleary et al., 2019).

PROMOTING THE INTERPROFESSIONAL TEAM IN HEALTH CARE

Individuals who work as a team need to prepare as a team. Continuing education for the entire team, not just individuals from various disciplines, provides professional development and is an investment in future success with predetermined patient outcomes. Also, ongoing professional development is important for fostering informed, accurate communication among team members and for continuity of care.

Recruitment of future professionals who want to be a part of team-based care needs to begin at the student level in each discipline. Maintaining ongoing relationships with interprofessional collaborative teams within precepting sites is crucial, as is building and sustaining relationships with clinical practices that serve as learning laboratories for interprofessional students. Rewards and incentives, such as attendance at professional development conferences and awarding stipends, help to recognize those sites and preceptors who demonstrate innovative health care (Nester, 2016).

NURSE LEADERSHIP, COLLABORATION, AND HEALTHY WORK ENVIRONMENTS

Healthy work environments and nurse leadership are mutually interdependent. In a systematic review of the literature regarding nursing workplace settings, Wei et al. (2014) cited the important role of nurse leaders in establishing healthy work environments, patient care quality, and evaluating nurse job performance. Equally, healthy work environments fostered nurse leaders' leadership capabilities.

Findings of the studies reviewed (Wei et al., 2014) indicated that nursing leadership and interprofessional collaboration are vital components of healthy work environments. These elements contribute to nurses' sense of fulfillment in their positions, as well as patients' satisfaction with the care they receive. Nursing leaders' abilities were positively associated with staff nurses' perceptions of the workplace atmosphere. Administrative support, too, was seen as a decisive factor in nurses' intentions to remain in their positions. Supportive leadership is fundamental in establishing healthy work environments, maintaining a stable nursing workforce, and promoting patient care quality. Also, a health-care organization's willingness to collaborate as part of a team effort is directly related to success or failure.

The systematic review (Wei et al., 2014) illustrates that a positive organizational culture and with a team focus of support and collaboration can lead to a healthy work environment. Equipped with a clear vision and mission, nurse leaders and administrators can empower staff to feel that they are part of a collaborative, interprofessional organization, thus transforming the workplace culture into one of innovation and caring at all levels.

Within the current complex health-care environment, no single individual or discipline is fully prepared to guide the many providers comprising the care team. Interprofessional teams will never replace the individual provider-patient relationship. Instead, this approach serves to enhance such a relationship, creating a more comprehensive, efficient, and personalized health-care experience. When promoted and nurtured, collaborative teams of clinicians and leaders can serve as powerful contributors to the success of patient health outcomes.

INTERPROFESSIONAL CARE TEAMS: KING'S THEORY OF GOAL ATTAINMENT

Imogene King's **theory of goal attainment** is a seminal work. In King's theory, health-care team decision making involves a process whereby the provider (nurse) and patient engage in mutual goal setting (King,1971). According to King, this is an interpersonal system involving four steps: (1) action, (2) reaction, (3) interaction, and (4) transaction. Within these steps, the nurse and patient share information about their perceptions, set goals through communication and interaction and agree on strategies to achieve these goals.

King stated that the goal of nursing is to help individuals to maintain their health so that they can function in their roles. The domain of the nurse includes promoting, maintaining, and restoring health and caring for the sick, injured, and dying. The function of a professional nurse is to interpret information in the nursing process to plan, implement, and evaluate nursing care.

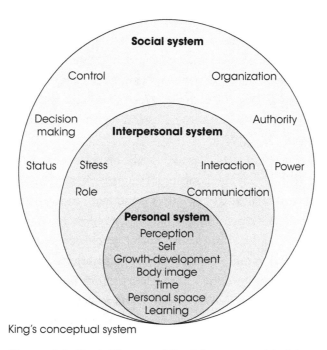

King's conceptual system

Figure 4.1 King's Theory of Goal Attainment Model

King gives detailed information about the steps of the nursing process in her model of nursing: assessment, nursing diagnosis, planning, implementations, and evaluation (King, 1990). Assessment occurs during interaction where nurses share specialized knowledge and skills, and patients share knowledge of their perceived issues. During the assessment, the nurse collects and interprets the patient data. Communication is required to verify the accuracy of the perception, as well as for interaction and translation (King, 1995).

The nursing diagnosis is developed using the data collected in the assessment. In the process of attaining goals, the nurse identifies problems, concerns, and disturbances about which the patient is seeking help. Following the nursing diagnosis, the nurse and health-care team collaborate to create a care plan of interventions to solve the problems identified. The planning is represented by setting goals and making decisions about the means to achieve those goals. This part of the transaction and the patient's participation are encouraged as a key to the decision-making process for determining how to achieve the stated goals (King,1995). The implementation phase of the nursing process involves actual activities performed to achieve the goals. In this model of nursing, it is the continuation of transaction.

Evaluation includes determining achievement of predetermined goals, as well as the effectiveness of nursing care. In a transactional process, communication must be reciprocal. King's theory can be applied to inform the design of a plan in which the interprofessional care team creates and maintains a patient-centered environment (King, 1990). To be successful in meeting patient outcomes, health-care providers (nurses, advanced practice nurses, physicians, physical and occupational therapists, and social workers) must frequently share and be mutually informed regarding relevant considerations. To guarantee optimal health care during the course of treatment, both the patient and provider/s must continually assess and adjust for changes in health, available resources, and gaps in care and treatments (King,1990).

King used the concept of *wholeness* to describe broader organizations and systems in which nurses work (King,1995). Her conceptual framework is organized into three systems: (1) personal, (2) interpersonal, and (3) social. A personal or individual system is essentially a single whole system, while an interpersonal system represents the interaction of two or more individuals in various environments. Social systems are composed of large groups, such as educational, community, or health-care organizations.

When goal setting involves the full participation of patients and health-care providers, where all participants agree on the means to achieve mutual goals, success is likely. The theory of goal attainment clarifies the nature of interprofessional collaboration. Application of the theory to inform the design of such collaboration increases the probability that collaborators' objectives will be attained. Integration of this theory into health-care fosters such collaboration with the expectation of improved patient outcomes (King, 1990).

SHARED GOVERNANCE

Shared, or professional, governance (Porter-O'Grady, 2017) is an essential foundation for nursing practice. Governance has grown from the established employee workgroup management structures similar to those in the corporate workplace. Nursing's current model reflects an understanding that the governing needs of a specific profession differ significantly from those of an employee workgroup. Nurses' governance relates to the best interests of those individuals they serve, as evidenced by comprehensive practice standards. These standards include knowledge generation and implementation, education and practice, quality indicators and competency requirements, ethics and disciplinary processes, licensure requirements, and professional behaviors (Clavelle et al., 2016; Crow & DeBourgh, 2017).

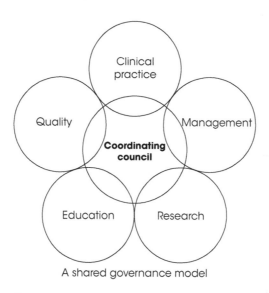

A shared governance model

Figure 4.2 Shared Governance Model

Health-care organizations have established shared/professional governance models within nursing organizations to create appropriate structures for governing the profession. Each considers organizational boundaries, administrative processes, leadership, and staff participation in shaping their professional governance models. In establishing governance models, many organizations examined those methods that would empower and engage nursing staff in their daily professional practices (Porter-O'Grady, 2019).

The standards that have surfaced are projected to represent critical concepts of professional governance. They provide a foundation on which to build sustainable models in all nursing environments. Three fundamental principles support these professional governance structures: (1) grounded in practicing nurse accountability, (2) built around accountability and clinical decision making, and (3) reflective of distributive decision making (Porter-O'Grady, 2019).

In the first principle (grounded in practicing nurse accountability), the professional takes personal accountability for ownership of any work. The nurse has an individual obligation to own and carry out those principles and practices associated with the profession. As a practice profession, nursing's goal is to positively affect patients' lives, accomplished through their own behaviors and based on principles established by their professional bodies (Porter-O'Grady, 2019).

The second principle (built around professional accountability and clinical decision making) involves those traditional organizations created around authority structures (Porter-O'Grady, 2019). In these models, workers are responsible for management-directed activities, where managers are accountable for the products of work. While this model is thought to advance productivity, professions, such as nursing, are different in that they are accountable to the populations they serve. Nurses own their decisions and actions, and they are personally answerable for the impact their actions have on those they help. It is the responsibility of the organization to design and maintain a management structure that supports both the profession's work and the accountability of each professional in the organization. Rather than a subordinate relationship of organization and profession, this plan signifies a collaborative partnership.

The third principle (reflective of distributive decision making) involves professional structures organized around decision making specific to each profession. Nurses are accountable for quality, competence, and knowledge needed to practice. In the past, this was considered part of the nurse manager's role. As a tradition that conflicted with the individual nurse's professional autonomy, this responsibility was no longer sustainable once the shared/professional governance model was introduced (Porter-O'Grady, 2019).

Applied appropriately and consistently, shared/professional governance structures provide support for incorporating quality, competence, and knowledge to transform professional nursing practice. According to Porter-O'Grady (2019), the journey continues. With millennials entering nursing, the demand for greater engagement and impact will grow. With nursing leaders informed regarding professional principles of governance and fairness, the greater the expectations for change will emerge.

Empowered and educated nursing leadership can end irrelevant, inefficient former practices. The creation of realistic, informed practice models to support professional nursing practice and advance collaborative partnerships is essential for sustainable, quality health care. With incorporation of the governance principles, partnered with accountable, equitable practices, and respectful behaviors among professional disciplines, the potential for transforming health care can be fully achieved.

EFFECTIVE COMMUNICATION TOOLS IN PROVIDING SAFE PATIENT CARE: THE HANDOFF REPORT

In today's complex health-care environment, hospitals are seeing an increased trend toward interdisciplinary care teams. This trend requires seamless collaboration and communication to ensure safe, optimal patient care (Cleary et al., 2019; Nester, 2016). As patient acuity and volume grow, it is essential for organizations to ensure that health-care provider teams have the necessary communication skills, policies, and procedures in place when transitioning patients between care settings.

Handoffs involve the transfer of essential information when the responsibility for care of the patient shifts from one health-care provider to another. When done effectively, there should be a seamless transition of critical information that results in continuity of patient care. During handoff, critical information regarding the patient's health is reported to the receiving provider. The type of information, communication methods, and variety of providers of patient care are a few factors that influence handoff efficiency and, as a result, impact patient safety. Time constraints require nurses to share essential information quickly, but the way this information is communicated varies. Also, information that one nurse may view as minor may be interpreted differently by another nurse.

The handoff between health-care providers is a key factor to fostering continuity in the provision of safe patient care. In their Sentinel Event Alert, the Joint Commission (TJC, 2017) raised concerns about the risks of handoffs, recommending that all hospitals develop a standardized approach to handoff communications. TJC reported that ineffective communication during patient handoffs remains a major contributing factor (70%) to various adverse events, such as wrong-site surgery, falls, medication errors, and delays in treatment. TJC indicated that communication errors resulted in more than 1,700 deaths and $1.7 billion in additional costs to the health-care system (TJC, 2017).

Successful handoffs must be standardized in content, forms, tools, and methods. During the handoff report, there should be opportunities to ask questions, methods to assess staff accountability, and ongoing education and mentoring. Also, the EHR should be used to enhance handoffs between senders and receivers (Agarwala et al., 2015).

THE SBAR (SITUATION, BACKGROUND, ASSESSMENT, RECOMMENDATION) HANDOFF

Sharing patient-specific, health-care information during the handoff requires situational awareness. **SBAR** is an effective communication tool for the patient handoff report. SBAR is a reliable, validated communication tool associated with a reduction in adverse events in hospital settings, improvements in communication among health-care providers, and promotion of patient safety (Shahid & Thomas, 2018).

SBAR was originally implemented in health-care settings with the intent of improving nurse-physician communication in acute care situations; however, it has also been shown to increase communication satisfaction among all health-care providers, as well as their perceptions that communication using SBAR is more precise. During handoffs, mnemonics such as SBAR may increase the memory of important steps and provide a structured and standardized process to follow.

The SBAR format provides a structured format for presenting patient information in a logical and succinct sequence; moreover, it is an efficient and intuitive tool to convey information to care providers. TJC (2017) described the SBAR as follows:

> *Situation: What is the situation?*
> *Background: What is the background information?*
> *Assessment: What is your assessment of the problem?*
> *Recommendation: How should the problem be corrected?*

Communication among interdisciplinary team members should be consistent, clear, and concise to make sure that all of the team members have an informed understanding of the patient's clinical information. The SBAR communication tool supports common language among team members, assists in shared decision making and conflict resolution among team members and ultimately improves patient satisfaction and outcomes. Shahid and Thomas (2018) reported that structured SBAR protocol for nurses' presentation of patient cases during interdisciplinary rounds resulted in shorter reporting times. In addition, SBAR provided an easy-to-follow linear format for the significant content nurses needed to convey to other providers of patient care.

I-PASS: ILLNESS SEVERITY/PATIENT SUMMARY/ACTION LIST/ SITUATION AWARENESS AND CONTINGENCY PLANS

Synthesis by Receiver

I-PASS is a multifaceted handoff improvement program that merges complementary interventions to improve handoffs and sustain these improvements over time (Starmer et al., 2017). As a structured approach to communication for patient transition, the mnemonic *I-PASS* stands for

> *Illness severity*
> *Patient summary*
> *Action list*
> *Situation awareness/contingency plans*
> *Synthesis by receiver*

Starmer et al. (2017) sought to determine the impact of a handoff improvement program for nurses by conducting a prospective pre-postintervention study on a pediatric intensive care unit. The intervention consisted of educational training, verbal hand-off I-PASS mnemonic implementation, and visual resources to provide reinforcement and sustainability. I-PASS implementation was associated with improvements in verbal handoff communications, including inclusion of illness severity assessment (37% preintervention vs. 67% postintervention, $p = 0.001$), patient summary (81% vs. 95%, $p = 0.05$), to-do list (35% vs. 100%, $p < 0.001$) and an opportunity for the receiving nurse to ask questions (34% vs. 73%, $p < 0.001$) (Starmer et al., 2017).

Implementation of the I-PASS Nursing Handoff Bundle was associated with wide-spread improvements in the verbal handoff process, without compromising nursing workflow. Nine medical centers employed the I-PASS system over the course of 10,740 patient admissions. Ultimately, preventable adverse events decreased by 30%, with a concurrent 23% reduction in medical errors. The program has since been adopted by more than 50 hospitals (Starmer et al., 2017).

BEDSIDE SHIFT REPORT (BSR)

Historically, the change-of-shift report took place at the nurses' station, away from patients. The change-of-shift report time was usually lengthy (up to an hour in some instances) with a rise in adverse events noted during this time period. Ofori-Atta et al. (2015) reported that the application of **BSR**, the change-of-shift report between nurses that occurs at the bedside, eliminates this gap in time and leaves the patient with a feeling of inclusion, as a partner in the plan of care.

With growing examination of patient safety issues in health-care delivery, health-care organizations sought to create a system based on current standards and best practices. TJC established a set of National Patient Safety Goals (NPSG) to improve the quality of care for patients. NPSG 2 involves improving the effectiveness of communication among caregivers, while NPSG 13 encourages patients' active involvement in their own care. The BSR meets both of these goals (2015).

Besides increasing patient satisfaction, compliance with these standards has also been shown to reduce costs to health-care facilities. Benefits include less paid overtime and decreased legal fees from falls and medication errors. According to Sherman et al. (2013), a significant bonus relates to improved patient experience survey scores from the Hospital Consumer Assessment of Healthcare Providers and Systems.

Once a hospital has identified targeted areas for improvement, staff participation, input, and acceptance of the creation and refinement of a standardized BSR is critical to eventual implementation (Ofori-Atta et al., 2015). Staff must receive orientation to the critical elements of BSR, which involves using the same language with introductions and with continuing the reporting process using SBAR. Also, patients and family, informed about BSR during the admission process, are provided with a consistent message, which fosters trust and compliance with the plan of care.

In their *Guide to Patient and Family Engagement*, the Agency for Healthcare Research and Quality (AHRQ, 2013) outlined the essential components of BSR:

- Introduce the nursing staff, patient, and family to one another.
- Invite the patient and (with the patient's permission) family to participate. The patient determines who is family and who can participate in BSR.
- Open the EHR at the bedside.
- Conduct a verbal report using the SBAR format in words the patient and family can understand.
- Conduct a focused assessment of the patient and a room safety assessment.
- Review tasks to be done.
- Identify the patient's and family's needs and concerns.

Because patients are made aware of the BSR during the admission process, they can be asked at this time about sharing information when visitors are present. If the patient wants complete privacy during this time, the nurse requests that visitors step out of the room to allow interaction between nurse and patient. Transparency is expected when it comes to patient safety. Initial efforts to replace an outdated reporting system may meet with challenges. However, it is anticipated that attitudes will change once measured, successful outcomes for patients, staff, and organizations are recognized (Ofori-Atta et al., 2015).

Reducing communication errors in all areas of professional practice can substantially improve patient safety and outcomes, quality of care, and satisfaction among health-care providers. As evidenced by the literature, there is a need for future research to assess the effect of a standardized handoff tool on patient outcomes, as well as cost-effectiveness, when compared to the occurrence of adverse events and communication errors. Studies on comparison and validation of the many communication tools employed in health care today, coupled with strategies to support the use of a standardized communication tool among health-care providers, are sorely needed.

Patient safety is a priority for inpatient care, and communication gaps are the most common cause of adverse events during patient care, despite the well-intentioned efforts of providers to avoid these errors during patient handoff. Employing an effective communication tool requires a significant investment of time for education and culture change for all involved to sustain clinical application. Future research is recommended to assess the validation and effect of current communication tools on patient outcomes in all areas of health-care delivery.

CHAPTER SUMMARY

In Chapter 4, the ADN to baccalaureate nursing student was introduced to the IOM Competency of Interprofessional Collaboration. Current nursing strategies to meet this competency were examined with examples provided by the inclusion of related literature. Challenges and benefits with incorporating the experience and expertise of a health-care provider team were explored in the efforts to effect successful completion of health-care outcomes for patients. Emphasis was placed on the concept of shared/professional governance and the need for nursing leadership and administrative participation in achieving positive change. The importance of early inclusion of interprofessional collaboration into nursing education's academic and clinical curriculum was supported with examples of current research in this area. Also, models of handoff communication were presented and compared to illustrate the collaborative efforts of providers to reduce medical errors and adverse events. The information disseminated in this chapter is intended to expand readers' knowledge and to inspire integration of the ideas and strategies presented into professional practice.

FOOD FOR THOUGHT: CRITICAL THINKING QUESTIONS

1. Describe a problem in your workplace. As a team leader, how would you organize, strategize, and collaborate with members of the health-care team to address the problem?
2. Identify those factors that can encourage or discourage interdisciplinary teamwork.
3. How do you assess and collect information on your patients (nursing process, systems model, other formats)? How do you prioritize the care of your patients?
4. What has been your experience with the concept of shared/professional governance? Cite examples.
5. What theories/theorists guide your practice as it relates to interprofessional teamwork?
6. What has been your experience with handoff communication tools, such as SBAR, I-PASS, BSR? Cite disadvantages and advantages.

SCENARIO: APPLYING WHAT YOU HAVE LEARNED

Interprofessional Collaboration and Delegation

Marianne, a veteran emergency department RN of 15 years, admits a client with a diagnosis of dehydration and heatstroke. Marianne completes an initial assessment of the client and assigns the physician's order of inserting an intravenous line to Ben, an

LPN who recently (within the last month) completed an IV therapy course approved by their state board of nursing regulations. Marianne offers to administer the normal saline intravenous solution when another nurse asks her assistance with an admission of a multiple trauma client. Although Marianne has not personally supervised Ben with this skill, she is aware of his proficiency in other nursing tasks. Ben assures Marianne that he is comfortable with the procedure. Marianne leaves to assist with the trauma case, asking to be notified immediately if problems occur.

Is it appropriate for the RN to delegate this task to the LPN? Why/why not? In answering this question, consider the following:

1. The client's diagnosis
2. The length of time the LPN has spent performing this procedure
3. The procedure itself
4. Staff involved
5. Potential complications
6. Approval from their state board of nursing regulations.

NURSING JOURNAL: REFLECT ON YOUR PRACTICE WHILE HONING YOUR WRITING SKILLS

Nurses as Agents of Change: Shared/Professional Governance

Change is a fact of life for nurses. From the technological advances that accelerate efficiency of care to assuming an evidence-based practice philosophy, nurses accept change. As a returning student, you see firsthand the outcomes of change in nursing and are prepared to meet the challenge by becoming an active participant in this transformation. You adapt to change day to day and perhaps minute to minute in some practice situations (Cleary et al., 2019)

When carrying out a change in your workplace, consider a shared/professional governance approach. Shared governance takes nursing quality improvement proposals from the bedside to the boardroom. It creates an opportunity for nurses to select changes that can improve patient outcomes, reduce health-care disparities, and advance health-care delivery.

- Consider a change you would like to make in your organization for this writing exercise.
- Will the change improve the clinical outcomes of your patient population?
- Will it allow you to track these outcomes?
- Will it help you more accurately identify areas for improvement?
- Will it increase the safety of care delivery?

- Will it make care delivery more efficient?
- Will it resolve process barriers?
- What resources will you identify?
- What are the time considerations for change to be implemented?
- What individuals will you involve in your plan for change?

As a coach in this endeavor, a positive change agent uses role modeling and mentoring to inspire members of the interprofessional team to adopt change. Change agents support and guide others toward successful program implementation in health-care organizations.

> You must be the change you want to see in the world.
>
> —*Mahatma Gandhi*

CHAPTER 4 REFERENCES

Agarwala, A. V., Firth, P. G., Albrecht, M. A., Warren, L., & Musch, G. (2015). An electronic checklist improves transfer and retention of critical information at intraoperative handoff of care. *Anesthesia & Analgesia, 120*(1), 96–104. https://doi.org/10.1213/ane.0000000000000506

Agency for Healthcare Research and Quality (AHRQ). (2013). *Guide to patient and family engagement in hospital quality and safety.* http://www.ahrq.gov/professionals/systems/hospital/engagingfamilies/guide.html.

American Nurses Association. (2015a). *American Nurses Association position statements on ethics and human rights.* www.nursingworld.org/MainMenuCategories/EthicsStandards/Ethics-Position-Statements

American Nurses Association. (2015b). *Code of ethics for nurses with interpretive statements.* www.nursingworld.org/MainMenuCategories/EthicsStandards/CodeofEthicsforNurses/Code-of-Ethics-For-Nurses.html

Arena R., & Lavie, C. (2015). The healthy lifestyle team is central to the success of accountable care organizations. *Mayo Clinic Proceedings, 90*(5), 572–576.

Clavelle J., Porter O'Grady, T., Weston, M., & Verran, J. A. (2016). Evolution of structural empowerment: Moving from shared to professional governance. *Journal of Nursing Administration, 46*(6), 308–312.

Cleary, M., West, S., Arthur, D., & Kornhaber, R. (2019) Change management in health care and mental health nursing. *Issues in Mental Health Nursing, 40*(11), 966–972. https://doi.org/10.1080/01612840.2019.1609633

Crow, G., & DeBourgh, G. (2017). Shared governance: The infrastructure for innovation. In S. Davidson, D. Weberg, T. Porter-O'Grady, & K. Malloch, (Eds.), *Leadership for evidence-based innovation in nursing and health* (pp. 401–437). Jones and Bartlett.

King, I. (1971). Toward a theory for nursing. In J. George (Ed.), *Nursing theories: The base for professional nursing practice* (pp. 26–27; 213–217). Appleton & Lange.

King, I. (1990). A theory for nursing: Systems, concepts, process. In J. George (Ed.), *Nursing theories: The base for professional nursing practice* (pp. 241–267). Appleton & Lange.

King, I. (1995). A systems framework for nursing. In M. McEwen & E. Wills (Eds.), *Theoretical basis for nursing* (pp. 173–177.). Lippincott Williams & Wilkins.

Institute of Medicine (IOM). (2011). *The future of nursing: Leading change, advancing health.* National Academies Press.

Nester, J. (2016). Importance of interprofessional practice and education in the era of accountable care. *North Carolina Medical Journal, 77*(2), 122–132. https://doi.org/10.18043/ncm.77.2.128.

Ofori-Atta, J., Binienda, M., & Chalupka, S. (2015). Bedside shift report: Implications for patient safety and quality of care. *Nursing, 45*(8), 1–4. *https://doi.org/10.1097/01.NURSE.* 0000469252.96846.1a

Porter-O'Grady, T. (2017). A response to the question of professional governance versus shared governance. *Journal of Nursing Administration, 47*(2), 69–71. *https://doi.org/10.1097/* NNA.0000000000000439

Porter-O'Grady, T. (2019). Principles for sustaining shared/professional governance in nursing. *Nursing Management, 50*(1), 36–41. *https://doi.org/10.1097/01.NUMA.0000550448.17375.28*

Rossler, K. L., Buelow, J. R., Thompson, A. W., & Knofczynski, G. (2017). Effective learning of interprofessional teamwork. *Nurse Educator, 42. https://doi.org/10.1097/NNE.0000000000000313*

Shahid, S., & Thomas, S. (2018). Situation, background, assessment, recommendation (SBAR): A communication tool for handoff in health care—a narrative review. *Safety in Health 4, 7.* https://doi.org/10.1186/s40886-018-0073-1

Sherman J., Sand-Jecklin, K., & Johnson J. (2013) Investigating bedside nursing report: A synthesis of the literature. *Medsurg Nursing, 22*(5), 308–312, 318.

Starmer A., Schnock, K., Lyons, A., Hehn, R., Graham, D., Keohane, C., & Landrigan, C. (2017). Effects of the I-PASS nursing handoff bundle on communication quality and workflow. *BMJ Quality & Safety, 6*(12), 949–957. http://dx.doi.org/10.1136/bmjqs-2016-006224

The Joint Commission (TJC). (2017). Inadequate handoff communication. *Sentinel Event Alert, 58,* 1–6. https://doi.org/https://www.jointcommission.org/assets/1/18/SEA_58_Hand_off_ Comms_9_6_17_FINAL_(1).pdf

Wei, H., Sewell, K. A., Woody, G., & Rose, M. A. (2014). The state of the science of nurse work environments in the United States: A systematic review. *International Journal of Nursing Sciences, 5,* 287–300. https://doi.org/10.1016/j.ijnss.2018.04.010

CREDITS

Employ Evidence-Based Practice

CHAPTER INTRODUCTION

In this chapter, the reader is introduced to the IOM core competency of evidence-based practice (EBP), its history, and its impact on the nursing profession and the delivery of patient care. The importance of possessinganEBP nursing philosophy is supported through examples, recent studies, and current literature.

KEY TERMS: MAKING CONNECTIONS

- IOM competency: evidence-based practice
- Clinical practice guidelines
- Critical thinking
- Evidence hierarchy
- Facilitator
- Iowa model
- Literature search
- PICOT
- Research

LEARNING OBJECTIVES/OUTCOMES

At the end of this chapter, students will accomplish the following:

- Trace the concept of EBP from its origins to its application in academic and practice settings in nursing today.
- Describe the components of the EBP process.
- Discuss how an EBP philosophy provides a foundation for lifelong nursing practice.
- Compare the relationships of critical thinking, clinical reasoning, and clinical judgment to EBP.
- Examine the implications of EBP for nursing from the perspective of research, best practice guidelines, evidence-informed practice, and technology.

Nurses are not just doers. Our work is supported by evidence and guided by theory. We integrate evidence and theory with our knowledge of patients and make important decisions with and for patients and families at the point of care. Research and practice are not separate but integrated. Nursing is a practice discipline with our own theories and research base that we both generate, use, and disseminate to others.

—*Antonia M. Villarruel, PhD, RN, FAAN Professor and Margaret Bond Simon Dean of Nursing*
University of Pennsylvania School of Nursing

A NURSE'S PERSPECTIVE

I have been an emergency room nurse for over ten years. My co-worker was caring for a 70-year old female patient experiencing an acute myocardial infarction (AMI), and I was helping him prepare the patient for a cardiac catheterization. It was a stressful situation and the patient was very upset. While my co-worker worked on the tasks needed to ready the patient for the procedure, I took her hand and spoke to her about her life, asking questions with the hope of distracting her while everyone worked around her. I spoke with her in a steady, quiet voice as though nothing was going on. I felt a rush of calm surround me in this moment. What she didn't know was that I was also counting her respirations, watching the pattern on her cardiac monitor and monitoring her state of alertness. From my experience and education as an ICU nurse, I knew that timely intervention and multitasking were essential. Despite years of evidence-based practice, I wondered if she would live to see the next minute of her life, let alone the next hour. Inwardly, I was panicking. What if she went into cardiac arrest? What if we couldn't save her? The calm that came to me in the midst of my inward panic actually came from talking to her and listening to what was important to her. Keeping her calm actually kept me calm.

I walked away from the cardiac catheter lab that day satisfied with the care that I had given. This is why I am an emergency room nurse: so that on what will prove to be the worse day of a patient's life, I can critically think through a situation. In the middle of the cacophony of alarms, pain of being poked and prodded, and the terror of being faced with death, I can help my patients by being physically, emotionally, and spiritually present. (RN to BS student)

EBP IN NURSING

The American Nursing Association Scope and Standards of Practice defines *the who, what, where, when, why, and how* of nursing practice (ANA, 2015). Integrated throughout the standards of practice is the viewpoint that EBP is key to the profession of nursing. Incorporating an EBP model into daily practice empowers nurses to make clinical decisions based on evidence from research, **critical thinking**, clinical expertise, and patient input.

EBP is the process of gathering, processing, and applying research outcomes to enhance practice, work settings, and patient outcomes. According to the American Nurses Association (ANA, 2015), nursing interventions should be practical, logical decisions based on EBP research studies. Using the EBP approach to clinical practice helps nurses provide high-quality, cost-efficient patient care. Through literature searches, examining data, and reviewing expert opinions, nurses can identify ways to provide quality, informed patient care (Stevens, 2013).

The EBP systematic process includes the following steps:

Ask a question.
Search the latest research.
Incorporate clinical experience.
Accommodate patient preferences.
Apply the results.

The impact of EBP has resonated across nursing practice, education, and science. The demand for evidence-based quality improvement and health-care transformation emphasizes the requirement for effective, efficient, and safe care. With the recommendations of national experts (IOM, 2001, 2010, 2011), nurses have presented contributions to fully deliver on the promise of EBP. Such initiatives have involved curricular restructuring, interdisciplinary collaboration, practice adoption, and scientific engagement in new fields of research (Stevens, 2013).

EBP IN NURSING: ORIGINS

The foundation of EBP has been traced to the1800s, with the work of Florence Nightingale. Credited with first evaluating and making decisions based on observed outcomes (Mackey & Bassendowski, 2016), Nightingale noted that unclean conditions and poor ventilation could negatively affect the health of patients. Specific instances of Nightingale's use of EBP included the practice of soap and water to clean skin, uncluttered environments, fresh air, light, and attention to patients' age and sex when providing care. Despite knowledge constraints at that time, coupled with the fact that the majority of medical decisions were made by male physicians, Nightingale was able to make changes and improve patient outcomes. She recorded medical statistics using patient demographics to determine the number of deaths in hospitals and mortality rates associated with different illnesses and injuries (Brower & Nemec, 2017).

The inception of EBP, actually termed evidence-based medicine, is credited to Archie Cochrane in the 1970s (Hulme, 2010). Bodies of research began to develop when it was discovered that physicians' decisions were often based on unfounded assumptions, leading to a diverse range of methods practiced by physicians for similar patient illnesses. Cochrane believed that physicians should carry out only those procedures that were considered effective (Cochrane Collection, 2013). Cochrane contended that randomized controlled trials (RCTs) offered the most reliable form of evidence. This belief provided a foundation of health-care decision making that evolved into the evidence-based medicine movement, which provided clinicians with the appropriate scientific evidence on which to base their clinical practice (Mackey & Bassendowski, 2016).

In their report, *Crossing the Quality Chasm*, the IOM (2001) urged all health professions to collaborate in the transformation of health care, proposing EBP as a solution to cross this chasm. Authorities continue to guide with successive IOM *Chasm* reports, with each version citing EBP as essential in closing the gap. The intent of EBP is to standardize health-care practices to reflect best evidence and to eliminate care disparities, leading to unpredictable and unsafe health outcomes. Consumer and professional demand for accountability in safety and quality improvement has further driven the need for implementing standardized EBP throughout health care (AHRQ, 2013; Mackey & Bassendowski, 2016).

LEVELS OF EBP: RATING SYSTEMS

As a problem-solving approach to clinical practice, EBP incorporates the best evidence from well-designed studies, patient preferences, and providers' expertise in making decisions about patient care. Levels of evidence-rating systems grade the quality of evidence generated from research. Acquiring knowledge about these levels is important to clinicians as they recommend or adopt a study, report, practice alert, or clinical practice guideline when making decisions about care (Dang & Dearholt, 2017; Glasofer & Townsend, 2019). A typical model describing the strength of evidence is an **evidence hierarchy**; this includes work from expert opinions and nonexperimental studies, to experimental investigations (Dang & Dearholt, 2017; Glasofer & Townsend, 2019). As the level of evidence advances up through the hierarchy, there is a greater probability of its use in guiding a health-care professional's practice decisions.

LOW LEVELS OF EVIDENCE involve expert opinions from observations of the health-care provider (Brower & Nemec, 2017). While they are to guide patient care in situations with limited research, there are risks in relying on personal observations. Examples of risks are assuming that a causal relationship exists (when in fact it does not) or the presence of conflicting expert opinions.

Viewed as more robust than expert opinions, MODERATE LEVELS OF EVIDENCE can be seen in nonexperimental studies, which are observational in nature and lack any manipulation of variables. Nonexperimental studies include longitudinal or cohort studies, designs investigating specific populations over time (Brower & Nemec, 2017). One such study example is weight gain in early adulthood and its possible link to health risks later in life, such as colon cancer.

The Framingham Study is widely recognized as the *gold standard* of longitudinal medical research. An original cohort of 5,209 subjects from Framingham, Massachusetts, between the ages of 30 and 62 years of age was recruited and followed up on for 20 years. The study listed various risk factors, such as advanced age, increased weight, tobacco smoking, elevated blood pressure and blood cholesterol, as well diminished physical activity. The Framingham Study's success stemmed from the fact that a large proportion of risk factors selected for analysis directly correlated with the development of cardiovascular disease (Dawber,1980).

Systematic reviews and randomized control trials comprise examples of HIGH LEVELS OF EVIDENCE. RCTs involve the arbitrary placement of a study population into two groups. One group is exposed to the research intervention, while the second, or control group, receives no intervention (Dang & Dearholt, 2017). A systematic review (SR) of RCTs analyzes the merits of individual studies and presents them as a collective whole to guide health-care practice. As a result, the conclusions of the SR can be used by organizations to develop health-care practice guidelines. Davenport et al. (2019) published an example of both an SR and a meta-analysis in their work involving the effect of prenatal exercise on maternal harm, labor, and delivery outcomes.

EVIDENCE HIERARCHY RATINGS

Level I: Experimental Study
RCT, SR of RCTs, with or without meta-analysis

Level II: Quasi-experimental Study
SR of a combination of RCTs and quasi-experimental, or quasi-experimental studies only, with or without meta-analysis.

Level III: Nonexperimental Study
SR of a combination of RCTs, quasi-experimental and nonexperimental, or nonexperimental studies only, with or without meta-analysis. Qualitative study or SR, with or without meta-analysis

Level IV: Opinion of Respected Authorities and/or Nationally Recognized Expert Committees/Consensus Panels Based on Scientific Evidence
Includes

- Clinical practice guidelines
- Consensus panels

Level V: Based on Experiential and Nonresearch Evidence
Includes

- Literature reviews
- Quality improvement, program, or financial evaluation
- Case reports
- Opinion of nationally recognized expert(s) based on experiential evidence

Source: Dearholt, S., Dang, D., & Sigma Theta Tau International. (2012). *Johns Hopkins nursing evidence-based practice: models and guidelines.* Sigma Theta Tau International.

IMPLEMENTING THE EVIDENCE
Incorporating EBP into health-care decisions can be completed at both an individual and organizational level. Ideally, both the provider and organization would support and work to incorporate evidence into health care. When organizations embrace EBP,

there is an associated increase in an individual's motivation to use research-proven practice (Kueny et al., 2015).

Research analyzing organizations that successfully use EBP report a culture that demonstrates originality and teamwork. Such an organizational EBP culture may have adopted a model of shared governance, such as the Magnet Recognition Program. This model focuses on advancing three goals within each magnet-designated organization: (1) promoting quality in a setting that supports professional practice, (2) identifying excellence in the delivery of nursing services to patients, and (2) disseminating best practices in nursing services (Broom & Tillbury, 2007). In addition, through the acquisition of online databases (Kueny et al., 2015), organizations invest in staff access to research and best practices. Other institutional approaches to support EBP include providing information technology workshops, as well as acknowledging staff members' professional development activities.

To facilitate EBP acceptance and maintenance, it is recommended that a unit **facilitator** be assigned (Kueny et al., 2015). Serving as a facilitator, an invested staff educator, manager, or an interdisciplinary team member would mean being available as a resource, presenting evidence at staff meetings, assisting with questions, and completing evidence reviews. Organizational support, such as funding reimbursement for EBP activities and attendance at conferences, can also foster implementation.

Most important to the acceptance of an EBP philosophy throughout an organization are the attitudes of health-care providers. Those professionals who question current practice, wonder if there are better answers, and strategize to find solutions and alternatives are more likely to investigate and conduct research. Also, they serve to inspire other members of the health-care team to follow suit.

HOW DOES EBP BENEFIT NURSES AND PATIENTS?

The inclusion of EBP in nursing provides nurses with the scientific research to make informed decisions. Through EBP, nurses remain current in their knowledge of guidelines and protocols for patient care. By searching for documented interventions, nurses can increase their patients' chances of recovery and future health. As part of an EBP practice philosophy, nurses include patients in the plan of care. Patients' proactive participation fosters active communication, compliance, and satisfaction with health-care decisions.

EDUCATING NURSING STUDENTS ABOUT EBP

In their educational curriculum, baccalaureate nursing students are provided with a fundamental introduction to and understanding of the research process in nursing practice. These programs cover the design, methodologies, process, and ethical principles of research. In addition, nursing students use critical thinking skills to evaluate and critique research studies to apply the findings to their nursing practice.

Nursing students recognize that through academic and clinical experiences, acquiring an EBP philosophy is essential to their chosen profession and lifelong learning. A valuable, problem-solving approach to clinical decision making, EBP integrates the best available scientific evidence with the best available experiential (patient and practitioner) evidence. EBP considers those internal and external influences on practice and encourages critical thinking in the application of evidence to the care of individual patients, families, and the community.

THE PICOT MODEL (POPULATION, INTERVENTION, COMPARISON, OUTCOME, AND TIME)

Searching for high-quality research data is a challenging and integral part of the EBP process. **The PICOT method** is a useful tool for providers as they identify a concept and create related key terms of interest. PICOT precedes a literature search as providers formalize themselves with the objectives of a proposed study. This method provides the user with the opportunity to produce a sentence replete with pertinent information. PICOT involves the population to be studied, the intervention or treatment, comparison of one intervention to another, the outcome anticipated, and the time element necessary to accomplish the outcome (Stillwell et al., 2010).

(P) PATIENT PROBLEM (OR POPULATION). Population refers to the sample of subjects you wish to recruit for your study. There may be a fine balance between defining a sample that is most likely to respond to your intervention and one that can be generalized to patients who are likely to be seen in actual practice. What are the patient's demographics, such as age, gender, and ethnicity? Or what is the problem or problem type?

(I) INTERVENTION. Intervention refers to the treatment that will be provided to subjects enrolled in your study. What type of intervention is being considered? Is this a medication of some type, or exercise, or rest?

(C) COMPARISON OR CONTROL. Comparison identifies what you plan on using as a reference group to compare with your treatment intervention. Many study designs refer to this as the control group. If an existing treatment is considered the "gold standard," then this should be the comparison group. Is there a comparison treatment to be considered? The comparison may be with another medication; another form of treatment, such as exercise; or no treatment at all.

(O) Outcome. Outcome represents the result you plan on measuring to examine the effectiveness of your intervention. What is the desired effect? What effects are not wanted? Are there any side effects involved with this form of testing or treatment?

(T) Time. What is the duration for your data collection?

The PICOT question format is a consistent "formula" for developing answerable, researchable questions. When you write a quality PICOT question, it makes the rest of the process of finding and evaluating evidence much more straightforward. A strong research question should always pass the "so what?" test. Who will the research help? What is the benefit? There should be a definitive and strong rationale for the purpose of the research. A well-thought-out, focused research question acts as the foundation of the study.

EXAMPLES OF PICOT QUESTIONS

P: For the population of nurses caring for preoperative surgical patients
I: Do formal preoperative nursing education sessions (perioperative process; medications, pain management; return to baseline level of daily activities, restrictions)
C: Current standard of practice (checklist)
O: Lead to reduced preprocedure anxiety, decreased recovery time in the Post Anesthesia Recovery Unit (PACU), improved patient perspective of total surgical experience?

P: In patients prescribed opiates for pain management
I: Does nursing education implementing complementary alternative medicine techniques
C: Compared to the use of prescribed opioids alone
O: Reduce patients' reports of level of pain, decrease their use of prescribed opioids, and minimize the potential for opioid addiction?

P: In hospitalized elderly patients with dementia or confusion
I: Do chair/bed alarms
C: Compared to 15-minute checks
O: Reduce the risk of falls
T: During length of stay?

READING AND CRITIQUING A RESEARCH ARTICLE

Nurses examine research data to find answers to their questions about best practices and to deliver quality, informed care. When choosing an article, it is important to first determine if it relates to a topic of interest or if it would be useful in clinical practice.

The following questions are intended as a guide to provide a fundamental framework for critiquing a research article.

- **Does the title accurately describe the article?** Titles will typically attract interest and provide an accurate description, but the article must first be read in its entirety. An informative title conveys the article's key concepts, methods, and variables.
- **Is the abstract representative of the article?** The abstract gives a brief overview of the study's purpose, research questions, methods, results, and conclusions. The information in the abstract helps the reader decide whether to continue reading the article.
- **Does the introduction make the purpose of the article clear?** An effective introduction provides the basis for the article. It includes a statement of the problem, a rationale for the study, and the research question/s. If there is a hypothesis being tested, it is stated clearly in the introduction and includes the anticipated results.
- **Is the literature review relevant to the study and comprehensive? Does it include recent research?** A literature review provides background information on the study. It establishes what information is known about the research problem. Most literature reviews include articles published within the previous 5 years. Seminal articles are influential or groundbreaking in literature reviews and may be included because of their historic value.
- **Does the methods section explain how a research question was addressed?** The methods section provides enough information to allow the study to be replicated. Components of this section indicate if the design is appropriate to answer the research question(s). Did the researcher select the correct sample to answer the research questions and was the size sufficient to obtain valid results?
- **How was data collected? Were the procedures listed in a step-by-step manner? Are the results presented clearly in the text and in tables and figures?** Results should be clearly summarized in the article's text, tables, and figures. Tables and figures are only a partial representation of the results, and critical information may be only in the text.
- **Are the limitations presented and their implications discussed?** Study limitations are important factors, as they inform why the results need further clarification, may only be generalized to certain situations, or may fail to provide anticipated results. Examples of limitations include poor survey response rates, or study participants who decline to be interviewed.
- **Does the discussion explain the results in relation to the theoretical framework, research questions, and significance of the study?** The discussion provides an opportunity to explain the results in respect to the research question/s. Authors use the

discussion section to interpret the results and explain the study's significance, as well as to provide recommendations for future research.

- **Is the study relevant to clinical practice?** Discuss whether the study will be useful in clinical practice.

LINKING EVIDENCE TO PRACTICE: THE CLINICAL PRACTICE GUIDELINE PROJECT

For EBP to be implemented, active engagement in reading, critiquing, and grading evidence must be considered a priority by all nurses in all situations. Equipping future nursing leaders with these transformative tools is an important first step. More than ever, health-care organizations today seek to employ nursing graduates who are empowered through education to critique existing practices and initiate evidence-based changes, resulting in better patient outcomes. This ability is a vital part of a nursing philosophy that focuses on evidence-based quality improvement. Also, state and national organizations are issuing credentialing directives and specifying that EBP in nursing is expected. Therefore, it is necessary to ensure that these aptitudes are firmly rooted in the education of nursing students (Heye & Stevens, 2009).

Although EBP is a well-known concept in the nursing profession, it has been observed that nurses continue to base their clinical decision making on past practice, as well as information from communication with colleagues, compared to searching nursing literature (Cronenwett et al., 2007). Compounding this problem is the disdain among some nursing students regarding research (Thornlow & McGuinn, 2010). Consequently, faculty teaching in undergraduate nursing programs face the challenge overcoming these behaviors through the creative integration of EBP content and competencies into their curriculum.

To inspire and prepare nursing students for quality improvement related to EBP, baccalaureate nursing faculty at a New England university examined their junior-level course's teaching and evaluation strategies for their research course, *Evidence-Based Practice in Nursing.* Upon review of the prospective research texts for the course, it was discovered that the content concentrated on competencies in research activities rather than the importance of research as a necessary tool for lifelong, evidence-based nursing practice. Faculty discussion and student feedback from prior course evaluations revealed that to relieve the uniform unfamiliarity and lack of interest regarding research among nursing students, course content should integrate strategies related to clinical practice. This feedback provided considerable insight into the preparation of nursing graduates. Expectations for new nursing graduates require EBP expertise for quality improvement in the present and future in the wake of complex care delivery systems. Students now must have experience navigating diverse information technology systems, as well as technical skill competencies for timely retrieval of the current, relevant information necessary to for the multifaceted care of patients (IOM, 2010).

With the goal of employing an interactive approach in teaching undergraduate nursing research, as well as aligning the curriculum to reflect the current AACN Essentials (2008), the course description was revised: "This course will introduce the student to the implementation of evidence based strategies. By the end of this semester, the student will be able to identify research processes, critique research studies and evaluate practice protocols" in furthering quality improvement. Also, course outcomes were modified to reflect the following skills acquisition by nursing students.

In the initial class meeting, junior baccalaureate students were introduced to the EBP course and given an overview of the content and expectations of the course. In this detailed review, course faculty provided an explanation of how concepts in each class built upon one another. The intent was to reinforce foundational knowledge from liberal arts and sciences and introductory nursing courses, clarify how course outcomes are threaded throughout the course and curriculum, and illustrate the course's alignment with the AACN Essentials (2008). The initial assignment, completion of a tutorial for National Institutes of Health certification on ethics in research, was presented at this time, geared toward educating students on the importance of the protection of subjects in research activities.

Prior to the beginning of the fall semester, a course faculty member met with nursing educators from the medical center where the baccalaureate students complete their clinical experience. The proposed objectives for a **clinical practice guideline (CPG)** project were presented to the nursing educators, who supported the idea and supplied the faculty member with CPG guidelines currently under review in their organization. The idea for a future forum during which students could exhibit their work to staff nurses in a poster presentation format was considered and a preliminary plan created (Illic & Rowe, 2013).

During the course introduction and overview, each assignment was outlined to 42 students enrolled in two sections. During the third class, students were divided into groups. Each group of four to five students was charged with selecting and examining a CPG. Subsequently, weekly classes were aimed at helping students build the following skills: develop a PICOT question, practice and refine foundational knowledge of literature searches and data retrieval, create a data search table, compare actual practice with evidence-based recommendations, and propose practice change based on gaps between actual practice and EBP.

The intent in creating the CPG project was to illustrate the value of supplemental learning tools in fostering nursing students' understanding and appreciation of an evidence-based professional philosophy, from knowledge development to application in practice improvement. Faculty anticipated that this strategy would validate the importance of actively linking research and practice. Increasing the abilities of nursing students in understanding EBP, national health-care improvement priorities, evidence-rating systems, and a model of knowledge transformation for EBP provided the inspiration for the project.

The following list of clinical practice guidelines were reviewed: catheter associated urinary tract infections, central line associated bloodstream infections, flushing of central lines, suicide prevention, hourly rounding to enhance fall prevention, and blind insertion versus X-ray confirmation for enteral tube feeding. Building on information from previous courses about the contribution of research to the discipline of nursing, initial class content incorporated fundamentals of conducting research, principles and design, sampling, and critique of quantitative and qualitative research. Permitting groups to select their clinical topic from the CPG "list" enhanced the relevancy of the project to their current clinical courses.

For students, a crucial component of the CPG project concentrated on framing a clinical question in preparation for performing a literature review. To foster this understanding, the PICOT model was used (Melnyk & Fineholt-Overholt, 2011). Problem-focused triggers can include clinical problems or risk management issues, while knowledge triggers might involve new research findings or clinical practice guidelines. Once the problem is identified and its importance established, the second step is to find, examine, and critique related literature. If enough evidence exists, the third step includes identifying research that supports a change in practice. Final steps involve effecting a change in practice and monitoring the outcomes. In the change process, Titler (2006) stated that commitment to EBP must be met at multiple system levels, from nursing staff through administration, suggesting that success lies in linking EBP and quality improvement initiatives.

THE LITERATURE SEARCH

A "library day" was scheduled during the fourth class to ascertain students' understanding of and skills in electronic database search strategies. During this time, the university librarian and faculty member assisted students with refining their PICOT questions, beginning their literature searches, and creating a data search table.

CRITICALLY APPRAISING THE EVIDENCE

The university's librarian proved to be an indispensable resource and inspiration to students with her hands-on approach to search strategies for locating and examining quality evidence. She developed a "library tutorial" unit on the course's Blackboard site and met with students multiple times over the course of the semester. Class discussion and a series of four short quizzes centered on assigned textbook chapters, as well as relevant readings (Melnyk et al., 2010). These activities were planned to ensure students' completion of required readings and reinforce understanding of the knowledge and skills needed to implement EBP consistently, one step at a time. In addition, rapid critical appraisals (RCA) of two scientific articles were assigned, with two class days spent examining this work. Prior to the due date, three lecture hours introduced concepts related to critical appraisal of research evidence. This was followed by a homework assignment in which students completed and submitted RCA "worksheets" in preparation for group discussion of the assigned activity.

Interactive class dialogue served to measure student understanding of the concepts surrounding critical appraisal of evidence. Group work gave students the opportunity to discuss the content of EBP in a less threatening atmosphere: a classroom of their peers. During discussions, students were engaged in helping, listening to, and learning from each other. In evaluation of this activity, students credited lecture, group work, and interactive discussion at each step of the article critique as efficient, effective ways of learning to critically appraise a scientific article.

COMPARING RECOMMENDATIONS TO ACTUAL PRACTICE: THE IOWA MODEL

The Iowa model (Doody, 2011) was incorporated into the students' presentation of their work. This exemplar highlights the importance of considering the entire healthcare system, from provider to patient to organization, using research within these contexts to guide practice decisions. A number of steps have been identified in the Iowa model to facilitate engagement in problem identification and solution development as they relate to incorporating evidence findings into practice. Developed by Titler and colleagues (2006), the model describes knowledge transformation and guides implementation of research into clinical practice. The seven steps identified here guide staff in the appraisal of evidence: (1) selection of a topic, (2) forming a team, (3) evidence retrieval, (4) grading the evidence, (5) developing an EBP standard, (6) implementing the EBP, and (7) evaluation (Doody, 2011).

EVALUATION

This capstone experience culminated in formal oral and PowerPoint presentations by each group at the end of the semester. Following the recommendations of Doody (2011) and Illic and Rowe (2013), in addition to the positive feedback from faculty, students applied and were invited to present their work as poster presentations at two events: Shared Leadership Day at the medical center and Annual Student Research Day at the university.

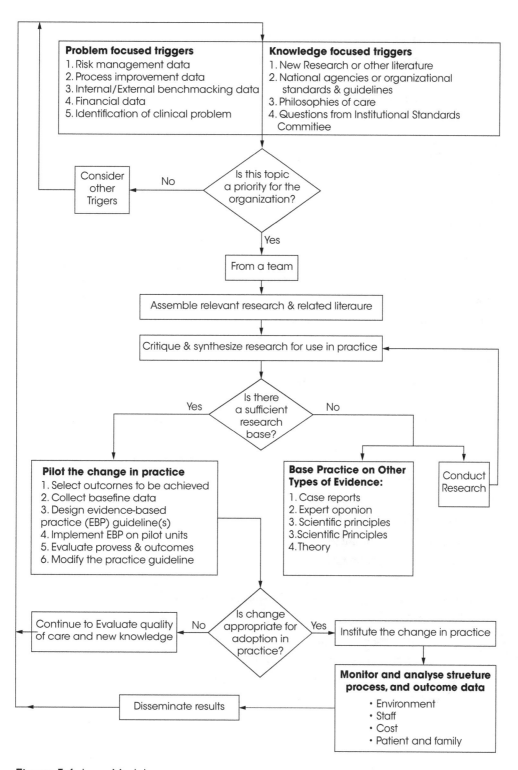

Figure 5.1 Iowa Model

Students' Evaluation of the CPG Project

Working collaboratively on this project provided an opportunity for students to discuss the significance, influence, and strength of the evidence supporting the recommendation to change health-care practice. Student presentations and faculty perceptions of the project indicated that beginning competencies in EBP were achieved.

IMPLICATIONS AND RECOMMENDATIONS

The CPG project proved to be an effective learning strategy. Through this process, students in the EBP class acknowledged the value of examining current, relevant literature. They developed an appreciation for the university's database resources, as well as the contributions of both nursing and multidisciplinary research for quality patient care. From this experience, students' recommendations included identification of hospital and nursing administration stakeholders to garner full support and encouragement in bringing the CPG project's recommendations to fruition, frequent interdisciplinary communication to keep the health-care team abreast of updates and changes, and ongoing staff in-services to focus on compliance with current guideline recommendations.

Students gained skills in reviewing evidence, classifying references, and applying data to recommend improvements in health-care practices. The project assisted students in recognizing the full process of change, from knowledge development to application in practice improvements. Collaborative experiential activities within student groups stimulated critical thinking and dialogue. Additional benefits occurred in informal meetings outside of class: conflicting ideas surfaced in groups and were referred to faculty for resolution and during the instructor's scheduled office hours where she discovered potential gaps in knowledge during significant intervals in student work and was able to intervene. Moreover, student groups acquired knowledge and experience of professional roles through poster presentations, peer review, and feedback. Expectations regarding professional dress and comportment conveyed the significance of formal collegial atmosphere, research, requirements for poster presentations, and the role of peer review.

Stevens (2013) reported that implementation of EBP is the nursing profession's best chance to reshape care that is safe, effective, and efficient. As the largest group providing care with the most patient contact, nurses have a significant opportunity to affect the course of illness and recovery. Therefore, nurses must actively engage in reading, critiquing, and grading evidence to continually challenge the profession. For EBP to be implemented, this value system must be considered a priority by all nurses in all situations. Equipping future nursing leaders with these transformative tools is an important first step.

IMPLICATIONS OF EBP FOR THE NURSING PROFESSION

It is vital that nurses be proactive in the pursuit of research knowledge to close the theory-practice gap. A study by Stokke et al. (2014) reported on the experience of EBP with 356 nurses. They found that the majority of nurses believe using EBP contributes to more positive outcomes for patients. However, many stated that they did not use evidence consistently and were less confident about its integration in practice.

Possessing and carrying out an EBP philosophy challenges nurses to be accountable and responsible for every action. At the core of nursing is patient-centered care, patient safety, and positive patient outcomes. With this in mind, nurses are challenged to comprehend and model EBP on a daily basis. In addition, nurses must work collaboratively within their health-care organizations and educational institutions to guarantee that current evidence encompasses all aspects of nursing care. Role modeling best practice guidelines, reviewing and implementing applicable research evidence, and taking advantage of technological advances are just a few actions to advance the nursing profession as a well-informed discipline into the future (Mackey & Bassendowski, 2016).

CHAPTER SUMMARY

In Chapter 5, the reader was introduced to the IOM Competency of EBP. Beginning with Florence Nightingale in the 1800s, EBP continues to advance within the discipline of nursing. EBP is foundational and provides a mechanism to minimize the theory-to-practice gap in the profession. This chapter discussed the concept of EBP from a historical perspective as it relates to nursing in the educational and practice domains. It is crucial that RNs be proactive in their quest for research knowledge so that the gap between theory and practice continues to close. Using nursing best practice guidelines, reviewing and implementing applicable research evidence, and taking advantage of technological advances are all ways in which nursing can move forward as a well-informed discipline.

FOOD FOR THOUGHT: CRITICAL THINKING QUESTIONS

1. What are the components of the EBP process?
2. How does EBP affect nursing practice, education, and research?
3. What is the relationship of critical thinking, clinical reasoning, and judgment to EBP?
4. What does EBP mean to you as a nurse? Give examples of how EBP serves as a foundation for your practice and a philosophy of lifelong learning.

SCENARIO: APPLYING WHAT YOU HAVE LEARNED

Critical Thinking and EBP

You are employed as perioperative assessment RN at a 950-bed medical center located in the northeast United States. Lawrence, a widowed, retired 70-year old, long-distance truck driver arrives for a preoperative assessment appointment and preoperative laboratory tests related to an upcoming knee replacement surgery. His additional diagnoses are hypertension, obesity, insulin dependent diabetes mellitus (IDDM), chronic knee pain and osteoarthritis of the left knee. Living alone on a farm 25 miles outside of a major city, Lawrence has always been independent. He has no living relatives. The nearest neighbor lives 5 miles away.

After surgery, Lawrence will be transferred to the subacute unit of the hospital for rehabilitation. He has been told by his orthopedic surgeon that, depending on his recovery, he should expect to remain in the hospital for 3–7 days. Lawrence states that he "will be fine" and "doesn't need any help once home."

In developing a plan of care for this patient, respond to the following questions:

1. What additional information do you need? Identify priorities.
2. Identify clinical guidelines/current research related to the perioperative experience that guides your approach.
3. Develop nursing diagnoses, short- and long-term goals.
4. Which interprofessional health-care team members should be involved in the plan of care?
5. What significant information must be included in a discharge teaching plan?

NURSING JOURNAL: REFLECT ON YOUR PRACTICE WHILE HONING YOUR WRITING SKILLS

Wonder Is the Beginning of Wisdom

1. From your nursing practice and from this chapter, identify a nursing-related topic/concept/problem you would like to investigate and explain why it is important to you.
2. From your identified concept of interest, develop a PICOT question. PICOT resources can be found in this chapter.
3. Conduct a literature search; locate a current scholarly nursing article (published within the last 5 years) regarding your concept and PICOT question.

4. Create a narrative about why you think this article is an example of scholarly best practice and how you would strategize its incorporation into your daily practice.

CHAPTER 5 REFERENCES

AHRQ. (2013). Agency for healthcare research and evidence for quality patient safety practices. *Making health care safer II: An updated critical analysis of the evidence for patient safety practices.* http://ahrq.gov/research/findings/evidence-based-reports/ptsafetyuptp.html

American Association of Colleges of Nursing (AACN). (2008). *The essentials of baccalaureate education for professional nursing practice.*

American Nurses Association. (ANA). (2015). *Nursing: Scope and standards of practice* (3rd ed.).

Broom, C., & Tilbury, M. (2007). Magnet status: A journey, not a destination. *Journal of Nursing Care Quality, 22*(2), 113–118. https://doi.org/10.1097/01.NCQ.0000263099. 21558.ec

Brower, E., & Nemec, R. (2017). Origins of evidence-based practice and what it means for nurses. *International Journal of Childbirth Education, 32*(2), 14–18.

Cochrane Collection. (2013). *Background of Cochrane.* http://www.cochrane.org/about-us/history/archie-cochrane

Cronenwett, L., Sherwood, G., Barnsteiner, J., Disch, J., Johnson, J., Mitchell, P., & Sullivan, J. W. (2007). Quality and safety education for nurses. *Nursing Outlook, 55,* 122–131.

Dang, D., & Dearholt, S. (2017). *Johns Hopkins nursing evidence-based practice: Model and guidelines* (3rd ed.). Sigma Theta Tau International.

Davenport,M., Ruchat,S., Sobierajski,F., Poitras, V., Gray, C E., Yoo, C., Skow, R. J., Garcia, A. J., Barrowman, N., Meah, V. L., Nagpal, T. S. …Mottola, M. F. (2019). Impact of prenatal exercise on maternal harms, labour and delivery outcomes: A systematic review andmeta-analysis. *British Journal of Sports Medicine, 53,* 99–107. https://doi.org/10.1136/bjsports-2018-099821

Dawber, T. R. (1980). *The Framingham study: The epidemiology of atherosclerotic disease.* Harvard University Press.

Doody, C., & Doody, O. (2011). Introducing evidence into nursing practice: using the IOWA model. *British Journal of Nursing, 20*(11), 661–664.

Glasofer, A., & Townsend, A. (2019). Determining the level of evidence: Experimental research appraisal. *Nursing Critical Care, 14*(6), 22–25. https://doi.org/10.1097/01.CCN. 0000580120.03118.1d

Heye, M., & Stevens, K. (2009). Using new resources to teach evidence-based practice. *Journal of Nursing Education, 48*(6), 334–339.

Hulme, P. A. (2010). Cultural considerations in evidence-based practice. *Journal of Transcultural Nursing, 21*(3), 271–280. http://tcn.sagepub.com/content/21/3/271

Illic, D., & Rowe, N. (2013). What is the evidence that poster presentations are effective in promoting knowledge transfer? A state of the art review. *Health Information and Libraries Journal, 30,* 4–12.

Institute of Medicine (IOM). (2001). *Crossing the quality chasm: A new health system for the 21st century.* National Academies Press.

Institute of Medicine. (IOM). (2010). *The future of nursing: Leading change, advancing health.* National Academies Press.

Institute of Medicine. (IOM). (2011). *The future of nursing: Leading change, advancing health.* National Academies Press.

Kueny A., Shever, L., Mackin, M., & Titler, M. (2015). Facilitating the implementation of evidence-based practice through contextual support and nursing leadership. *Journal of Healthcare Leadership, 7,* 29–39. https://doi.org/10.2147/JHL.S45077

Mackey, A., & Bassendowski, S. (2016). The history of evidence-based practice in nursing education and practice. *Journal of Professional Nursing, 33*(1), 51–55. https://doi.org/http://dx.doi.org/10.1016/j.profnurs.2016.05.009

Melnyk, B., Fineholt-Overholt, E., Stillwell, S., & Williamson, K. (2010). The seven steps of evidence-based practice. *American Journal of Nursing, 110*(1), 51–53.

Melnyk, B., & Fineholt-Overholt, E. (2011). *Evidence-based practice in nursing and healthcare: A guide for best practice* (2nd ed.). Lippincott.

Stevens, K. (2013). The impact of evidence-based practice in nursing and the next big ideas OJIN. *The Online Journal of Issues in Nursing, 18*(2), Manuscript 4. https://doi.org/10.3912/OJIN.Vol18No02Man04

Stillwell, S., Fineout-Overholt E., Melnyk, B., & Williamson, K. (2010). Evidence-based practice, step by step: Asking the clinical question: A key step in evidence-based practice. *American Journal of Nursing, 110*(3), 58–61. https://doi.org/10.1097/01.NAJ.0000368959.11129.79

Stokke, K., Olsen, N., Espehaug, B., & Nortvedt, M. (2014). Evidence-based practice beliefs and implementation among nurses: A cross-sectional study. *BMC Nursing, 13*(1), 8. https://doi.org/10.1186/1472-6955-13-8

Thornlow, D., & McGuinn, K. (2010). A necessary sea change for nurse faculty development: Spotlight on quality and safety. *Journal of Professional Nursing, 26*(2), 71–81. https://doi.org/10.1016/j.profnurs.2009.10.009

Titler, M. (2006). Developing an evidence-based practice. In G. LoBiondo-Wood & J. Haber (Eds.), *Nursing research: Methods and critical appraisal of evidence-based practice* (6th ed.), 385–437. Elsevier/Mosby.

CREDIT

Apply Quality Improvement (QI)

CHAPTER INTRODUCTION

In this chapter, the reader is introduced to the IOM Competency of Quality Improvement (QI) in which individuals collaborate to refine outcomes in the improvement of systems, leading to an enhanced patient experience, improved overall population health, and reduced costs of care. Lewin's model of change theory, the Lean model, and QSEN are presented as examples of patterns of change for safe QI in health care. Examples from practice and literature are incorporated into each section of the chapter to inform and support learning and enhance professional practice.

KEY TERMS: MAKING CONNECTIONS

- Blame-free work environment
- Just culture of safety
- Lewin's change theory
  - o Unfreezing
  - o Change
  - o Refreezing
- Lean model
- Plan-do-study-act (PDSA)
- Quality improvement (QI)
- QSEN
  - o Knowledge

- o Skills
- o Attitudes
- Root cause analysis
- Walk arounds

LEARNING OBJECTIVES/OUTCOMES
At the end of this chapter, students will accomplish the following:

- Examine how the IOM reports on quality care have affected nursing and the delivery of health care.
- Describe Lewin's change theory and its relevance to nursing practice.
- Discuss the importance of integrating quality and safety competencies into nursing practice.
- Identify the four steps of quality improvement.
- Review the PDSA cycle and its usefulness in QI.
- Characterize priorities for addressing the current state of patient and workforce safety.

It is not the strongest of the species that survives, nor the most intelligent, but the one most responsive to change.

—*Charles Darwin*

The secret of getting ahead is getting started. The secret of getting started is breaking your complex overwhelming tasks into small manageable tasks, and then starting on the first one.

—*Mark Twain*

A NURSE'S PERSPECTIVE

I started my career as a certified nurse's aide, then moved on to a licensed practical nurse program at a local community college. I completed the program and bridged into my second year of the community college's registered nurse program the following fall. I graduated and was planning on returning for my baccalaureate degree; however, health issues got in the way. I am happy to say I am healthier now and ready to tackle this program! Change is good. I hope that I can take away knowledge and skills that will help me become a stronger nurse in the working field. I have always tried to be the best nurse I can be, and my end goal is to have the initials "BSN" after my name. (RN to BS student)

LEWIN'S CHANGE THEORY

Regarded as one of the modern pioneers of social, organizational, and applied psychology in the United States, **Kurt Lewin developed change theory** (Lewin, 1951). His model represents a dynamic balance of forces working in opposing directions and includes three key concepts: (1) driving forces, (2) restraining forces, and (3) equilibrium. These driving forces create a *push-pull* effect as an individual navigates through the process of change.

Restraining forces are those life experiences that oppose change (fears, threats), while driving forces inspire change (personal goals, career advancement). While driving forces steer individuals in a desired direction, causing a shift in the equilibrium toward change, restraining forces hinder change by sending individuals in the opposite direction. Equilibrium is a state of being where driving forces equal restraining forces. It is a condition where no change occurs but can be raised or lowered by changes occurring between the driving and restraining forces (Lewin, 1951; Shirey, 2013; Wojciechowski et al., 2016).

UNFREEZING, CHANGE, AND REFREEZING

Lewin's most influential theory was his model of the change process in human systems. He theorized a three-stage model of change that is known as the *unfreezing-change-refreeze* model that rejects and replaces prior learning. The method involves preparing individuals for change, making those changes, and, finally, integrating and normalizing those changes within the organization (Lewin, 1951).

Unfreezing involves the tendency of individuals to seek out an environment of relative safety to maintain a sense of control. Attaching their sense of identity to their environment creates stability for individuals from which any alternatives, even those that may offer significant benefit, will cause discomfort. Talking about the future will not necessarily transfer individuals from a *frozen* state. Substantial effort may be needed to *unfreeze* and motivate individuals for readiness to change. Some individuals are *change ready*, while others may need more to leave their comfort zones (Shirey, 2013).

Change focuses on the belief that change is a journey rather than a simple step. Change is difficult and requires considerable time and support. A typical barrier occurs when leaders spend time with their own personal journey, assuming that others should automatically follow suit. For many, the hardest part of this stage is in beginning the change. Individuals can become caught

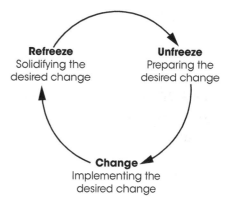

Figure 6.1 Lewin Model

in situations where they are not accountable for the risks of work in transitioning and where talking about change is substituted for action (Shirey, 2013).

Refreezing entails putting down roots again and establishing a new place of stability. This stage is often rather tentative and can lead to a state of *slush*, where freezing is never attained. *Change shock* occurs, in individuals working at low levels of productivity while waiting for the next change (Shirey, 2013).

THE LEAN MODEL

The Lean systems approach (LEAN) focuses on supporting individuals through a standardized system of work to improve process flow and to highlight inefficiencies, with the intent of empowering staff to take action on all levels. The goal of the lean process is to eliminate waste in areas such as time, inventory, overproduction, and transportation.

In a case review, Wojciechowski et al. (2016) describe how a large Midwestern rehabilitation hospital developed an intervention model for implementing and maintaining bedside shift reporting. The project demonstrates that many disciplines can employ common frameworks, such as Lewin's three-step model for change and the lean systems approach, to lead change, support outcomes of high-quality and safe care, and to capitalize on the benefits of different viewpoints and discipline-specific approaches.

The lean system represents a culture in which each staff member is encouraged to contribute to change. The model emphasizes creating value, supporting staff, and improving process flow to increase quality, reduce costs, and increase efficiency. Interprofessional collaboration involves making improvements to observe, ask questions, and learn. Other aspects of lean include using data and employing root cause analysis to solve problems (Wojciechowski et al., 2016).

Evolving as a learning organization by creating a safe, blame-free environment to make mistakes (while respecting patient safety) is a major component of lean. This model employs a philosophy that it is better to try, fail, learn, and adjust than not to try at all. With lean, staff can break down problems, eliminate ineffective activities, and establish a foundation for building a safe, positive work environment (Wojciechowski et al., 2016).

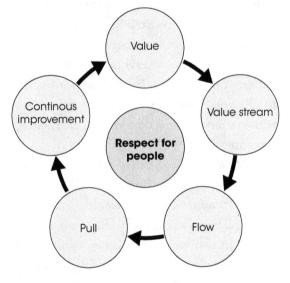

Figure 6.2 LEAN Model

Integrating concepts from both Lewin's three-steps for change and the lean systems approach uses the best of each method to maintain interprofessional collaboration using a problem-solving approach. Through this approach, nursing and other disciplines can continue to improve outcomes for the greater good of patient outcomes and health-care organizations. While Lewin's theory provides fundamental principles for change, the lean system provides aspects of accountability, communication, employee engagement, and transparency to develop and implement change (Wojciechowski et al., 2016).

QI

Florence Nightingale predicted that change was essential for nursing to thrive. Nightingale set the vision for nursing as a profession by establishing principles and priorities for nursing education. A leading proponent of evidence-based care, Nightingale advocated for integrating interprofessional learning systems to continually improve the health of patients. She encouraged hospital leaders to embrace patient and workforce safety as essential standards in their organizations (Maindonald & Richardson, 2004).

Interpreting and disseminating data are essential for improvement. Nightingale called statistics "the most important science in the world." Her **root cause analysis** showed that British soldiers were more likely to die from the spread of typhoid, cholera, and dysentery because of unsanitary conditions than their battle injuries (Maindonald & Richardson, 2004). On the anniversary of her 200th birthday (May 12, 2020), we celebrate Nightingale's many advances and accomplishments in the area of continuous **quality improvement**.

Embracing change at the core of nursing and health care is a challenge, as many in this population are resistant to change and cling to old patterns of behavior. Part of the challenges and strategies faced in the profession are related to the movement of information and knowledge from the point of research to implementation of evidence-based best practice. Nurse leaders' endorsements of change management principles and strategies will help to steer and to grow the developments that have changed nursing in such a short period of time (Cleary et al., 2019).

Continuous QI is a concept that includes the following aspects: quality assurance, which provides services to meet an appropriate standard; problem resolution, which includes departments involved in a particular issue; and QI, an ongoing process, which involves all organizational levels collaborating to produce better services for patients. Those providers who perform direct services are in the best position to identify the need for change in service delivery processes. QI uses data to examine outcomes of care processes and improvement methods. The information obtained is used to design and test changes for continuous improvement of the quality and safety of health-care systems (Dolansky & Moore, 2013). The QI process models a *blame-free* environment by creating a system that prevents errors and improves health outcomes.

QI projects typically involve a team process. Whether an organization is seeking to improve patients' satisfaction with specific care needs and wait times or interpreting their providers' explanations, a team approach helps an organization to achieve significant and lasting improvements. Each individual team member is an active and contributing participant, bringing unique perspective to the process. Contributions are made from each individual's skill set and the team's synthesis of ideas (Health Resources and Services Administration [HRSA], 2011).

Nurses, who are at the heart of the system, are well qualified to assess the status of health-care services and to work toward improving the processes by which these services are provided to clients in the health-care setting. Nurse management can structure the work setting to foster staff's ability to undertake constructive action for improving care. The use of QI forums to facilitate the coordination of QI efforts is an effective way to achieve success.

By inspiring and empowering nursing staff in their efforts to improve the process by which health care is provided, nurse managers participate in reshaping the health-care environment. The professional nurse plays a vital role in the QI of health-care services. However, nurses cannot make these improvements in a vacuum. Total quality commitment must include all levels of an organization's structure. Quality patient care services will be achieved as the result of positive interactions among departments working together to build a dynamic mechanism that continuously improves the processes and outcomes of health-care services.

During an ongoing QI program, the team may think they are accomplishing little. Applauding each success, no matter how minor, helps to overcome that feeling. QI is challenging work, and celebrating progress can break the routine and inspire further creativity. Also, taking the time to document a team's achievements makes it easier to recall accomplishments when writing grant proposals (HRSA, 2011).

THE FOUR STEPS OF QI
(Based on information from Famolaro et al., 2016)

1. **Identify: Determine what we want to improve**
    The first step of QI is initiated with the realization that there is a need for improvement. A patient might question the quality of care provided or an adverse event signals a process that is problematic. The questions below assist with identifying a problem:

    • What is the problem?
    • How do you know that it is a problem?

- How frequently does it occur, or how long has it existed?
- What are the effects of this problem?
- How will you know when it is resolved?

2. **Analyze: Understand the problem**

   The second step of QI identifies the opportunity for QI. Analysis examines the process to be improved or the system. Outcomes here involve include explaining why the process must be improved, measuring process performance to create the effect, and articulating research questions (below). To meet the outcomes, this stage involves the use of data.

- Who is involved or affected?
- Where does the problem occur?
- When does the problem occur?
- What happens when the problem occurs?
- Why does the problem occur?

3. **Develop: Hypothesize about what changes will improve the problem**

   The third stage is activated with sufficient collection of data is in place. A hypothesis is created regarding those interventions to mitigate the identified problem.

4. **Test/implement: Test the hypothesized solution to see if it yields improvement. Based on the results, decide whether to abandon, modify, or implement the solution**

   This stage involves testing and implementation of the hypothesis, known as the **plan-do-study-act (PSDA)** cycle. The extent of this stage depends on the size and complexity of the QI plan.

MODEL FOR IMPROVEMENT: PDSA

Once a team has set an aim, established its membership, and developed measures to determine whether a change leads to an improvement, the next step is to test a change in the real work setting. The PDSA cycle is shorthand for testing a change by planning, trying, observing the results, and acting on what is learned. Similar to the nursing process of assessment, diagnosis, plan, intervention, and evaluation, this method is considered helpful for all health-care providers for action-oriented learning and continuity of care (American Society for Quality, 2009).

Table 6.1 PDSA Model

1.	**Plan**	Collect baseline data to measure the effects of change. Plan to monitor the effects of change through a data collection system. Educate and communicate with others about the change. Inform and include people involved in the change and make sure they accept it.
2.	**Do**	Test the change (intervention). Verify that the change is being implemented as planned. Collect data about the process being changed. • Check that the data are complete. • Document any changes not included in the original plan.
3.	**Study**	Verify that the change was implemented according to the plan. See if the data are complete and accurate. Compare the data with the baseline information to look for an improvement. Compare predicted or desired results with the results from the test.
4.	**Act**	Summarize and communicate what was learned from the previous steps. If the plan does not yield the desired results, modify or abandon the plan and repeat the PDSA cycle if necessary. Implement the change as standard procedure if it proved to be successful. Monitor the change over time to check for improvements and problems.

EXAMPLE OF A TEST OF CHANGE (PDSA CYCLE)

Depending on their aim, teams choose promising changes and use PDSA cycles to test them quickly on a small scale, see how they work, and refine them as necessary before implementing the changes on a broader scale. The following example shows how a team started with a small-scale test.

LACTATION MANAGEMENT TEAM, POSTPARTUM BREASTFEEDING MOTHER

Planned Visits for Breastfeeding Assistance

Plan. Team of maternal child health nurse and lactation consultant ask patient if she would like more information on/assistance with breastfeeding techniques and problem management.

Do. Team conducts patient interview and assessment.

Study. Patient conveys interest; team pleased at patient's positive response.

Act. Nurse/lactation consultant will set up a planned visit in 2 days.

Objective: PDSA *Teach Back Method* to Improve Patient Understanding of Care Plan

- **Plan.** With the mother of a newborn, the nurse will assess knowledge level using the *teach back* method

- **Do.** The nurse attempted teach back regarding newborn care with her assigned postpartum patient. She discovered that her patient needed help with breastfeeding positions and bathing techniques for her newborn. The nurse was able to show the patient different feeding positions and demonstrated a newborn bath. The patient asked appropriate questions and verbalized understanding. Also, the patient completed a *return* newborn bath demonstration. The nurse reported confidence in the patient's skills.

- **Study.** The nurse recognized the assumptions she had been making. This was the mother's second child, but her first born child is now 12 years old. In addition, the patient is new to the community and lives several hours away from family and friends. Her single support system is her husband, who is employed as a long-distance trucker and travels out of state each week.

- **Act.** The nurse recognizes the need to involve social services and the local visiting nursing agencies to provide resources and support for the patient. Written instructions and contact information for the Visiting Nurses Association (VNA), Women, Infants and Children (WIC) office, La Leche League (breastfeeding support), lactation counselor, and the local mothers support group were provided. Upon discharge, the nurse schedules for her patient the following appointments: pediatrician, obstetrician, and home visits from VNA, WIC, and lactation counselor.

Source: American Society for Quality. (2009). Project planning and implementing tools: Plan-do-check-act cycle. http://www.asq.org/learn-about-quality/project-planning-tools/overview/pdca-cycle.html

Doerner and Swenty (2019) designed a QI project to evaluate the effectiveness of a perioperative *clinical immersion* experience on the perceptions of readiness for practice held by senior nursing students working toward a baccalaureate degree. Seven senior nursing students participated in the experience. Following the clinical immersion, participants were interviewed to determine their perceptions. Data analysis and identified recurring key words were evaluated further as attributes of critical thinking, skill competency, and role socialization. Findings revealed students' positive perceptions of growth and readiness for practice.

This valuable clinical opportunity immersed student participants into a highly specialized professional nursing setting and enhanced their understanding of the perioperative nursing role. More importantly, the experience afforded participants possible employment (following graduation and successful completion of the National Council Licensure Examination (NCLEX) in a professional practice as a perioperative nurses (Doerner & Swenty, 2019).

Nurses play a vital role in the QI of health-care services. However, they cannot make these improvements in a vacuum. Total quality commitment must include all levels of an organization's structure. Quality patient care services will be achieved as the result of positive interactions among departments working together to build a dynamic mechanism that continuously improves the processes and outcomes of health care services.

QSEN

In response to calls for improved quality and safety (IOM, 2003), leaders from schools of nursing across the United States created the **QSEN** initiative. Funded by the RWJF, six QSEN competencies were established with KNOWLEDGE, SKILLS, AND ATTITUDE statements for each competency. The goal of the QSEN initiative is to create an association of health-care providers who contribute to a culture of quality and safety. The ultimate goal is to coordinate quality and safety education, scholarship, and resources (Cronenwett et al., 2007).

Competency statements are the tools nurse educators and clinicians use to identify curricular gaps so that changes to incorporate quality and safety education can be made (Barnsteiner et al., 2013). The QSEN website (https://qsen.org/about-qsen/), is a national educational resource for nurses and encourages the distribution of research related to teaching strategies aligned with QSEN's six competencies of patient-centered care, EBP, teamwork and collaboration, safety, QI, and informatics (Dolansky & Moore (2013).

QSEN 's greatest challenge is to provide nurses with the knowledge, skills, and attitudes to continuously improve the quality and safety of their workplaces. This charge includes specific competencies to ensure that quality and safety standards are not only achieved but also continuously improved. Each competency integrates the **knowledge, skills and, attitudes** nurses should possess in providing informed care. In the **knowledge** component of the patient-centered care competency, nurses examine barriers that deter patients' participation in their care. The **skill** component of the plan eliminates barriers and provides access to appropriate resources. The **attitude** component takes place when nurses are empathetic to and understanding of individual patient needs and preferences for carrying out the plan of care.

QSEN competencies empower nurses to hold themselves to high standards when working with their patients while also encouraging them to use critical thinking and problem-solving skills. New nurses often go through a minimum of a weeklong orientation with demonstrations and tests to validate competencies taught in school. Within this orientation process, quality and patient safety are integrated. Quality and safety in education are continual learning processes for nurses. Best nursing practices incorporate QSEN competencies as, ultimately, these competencies save lives.

A JUST CULTURE OF SAFETY

The term **just culture** refers to a system of shared accountability in which organizations are answerable for the systems they have designed and for the behaviors of their employees, in a fair and just manner. Employees are accountable for the quality of their choices and for reporting errors. Creating a safe, transparent, **blame-free working environment** encourages reporting of mistakes and hazards and, ultimately, improves patient care (Famolaro et al., 2016).

In order to create a culture of justice and safety, hospital organizations must ensure that staff are treated fairly when involved in an adverse event. Both the Agency for Healthcare Research and Quality (AHRQ) and TJC define patient safety culture as the degree to which an organization's beliefs, values, and norms encourage patient safety. A **culture of safety** encompasses all levels of a hospital system, where leaders support the actions of staff throughout the organization (Famolaro et al., 2016).

TJC (2009) lists the following traits of a safety culture:

- Staff and leaders value transparency, accountability, and mutual respect.
- Safety is everyone's first priority.
- Behaviors that undermine a culture of safety are unacceptable.
- Staff recognize that systems have the potential to fail and are, therefore, mindful of identifying hazardous conditions and close calls before a patient is harmed.
- Staff report errors because they know the information can be used to address system flaws that contribute to patient safety events.
- Staff create a learning organization by learning from patient safety events to continuously improve.

Leadership backing of a safety culture must demonstrate the type of behavior expected from staff to support such a culture. The Emergency Care Research (ECRI) Institute, a federally certified patient safety organization, encourages patient safety **walk**

rounds by administration and staff to demonstrate a commitment to safety Emergency Care Research Institute (ECRI), 2019). The process involves organizational leaders visiting various areas of the hospital on a regular basis, interviewing providers and frontline staff, and asking specific questions about patient safety.

A culture of safety encourages individuals to voice their concerns about issues that could jeopardize patient safety. A just culture recognizes that human beings are fallible, particularly in workplaces where the system is flawed. Contrary to this, a shame and blame environment brings error reporting to a halt. Individuals in these environments are reproached for mistakes that may have deeper safety concerns. Without the information from an error report, there can be no learning from the adverse event (Leonard & Frankel, 2010).

Fundamental to a safety culture is an organization's willingness to examine its own weaknesses by conducting a **root cause analysis** and using the findings to improve care delivery. High-reliability organizations create and maintain a high level of safety by demonstrating a proactive stance to learn and change before accidents occur. Using event reporting programs, they look for, identify, and fix problems before harm can occur. When adverse events do occur, high-reliability organizations investigate them to identify and address the underlying system faults that contributed to the problem.

CHAPTER SUMMARY

In Chapter 6, through examination of the IOM Competency of QI, examples from the literature, practice, and various models, readers were reminded of the importance of change for personal and professional development, as well as for continual learning, in the pursuit of quality, informed, and safe patient care. Recognition of the need for all health-care providers to work as an interprofessional team in recognizing problems and maintaining transparency in professional practice in the pursuit of a culture of safety was emphasized and supported by the current research cited in the chapter.

FOOD FOR THOUGHT: CRITICAL THINKING

1. What QI projects have you seen, heard about, or learned about, and what are the expected or desired outcomes?
2. How would you describe the culture of safety and a "blame-free" environment in your workplace?
3. Can you identify common workplace safety issues and how they are managed on your unit?
4. Examine how the IOM reports on QI have affected nursing and health-care delivery.

SCENARIO: APPLYING WHAT YOU HAVE LEARNED

Quality Improvement

As an ADN with seven years' experience, Jillian has spent most of her previous career working on the subacute unit. Three years ago, Jillian enrolled part time in an ADN to BSN nursing program at a local university. She recently graduated with honors. Jillian has been hired as an evening (3:00 to 11:00 p.m.) staff RN on the same medical surgical unit.

Jillian is now engaged in a six-week hospital/unit orientation and has maintained a positive working relationship with her preceptor. The preceptor has been assigned consistently to Jillian for 1 month; however, because of to a medical emergency, her preceptor has not been available during the last week.

Jillian was informed that for the rest of her orientation, she will have a new preceptor. The new preceptor admits to Jillian that she was "assigned" to the preceptor role and is not happy about the "extra work" involved. She also has voiced her opinion that "there is no way you can get a BSN in that short amount of time. What kind of a program are they running over there at the university?" Although she is still on orientation, Jillian is left alone to make her own decisions.

A conflict occurs when Jillian overlooks a client's confusion and fall as a result of a newly prescribed medication. Her new preceptor angrily admonishes Jillian at the nurses' station. Jillian feels overwhelmed and defeated and is thinking she should resign from the position: "Maybe my nursing program did not prepare me … maybe my original preceptor was too easy on me."

Scenario Questions

How could this situation have been avoided?
What strategies should be in place at this time?
What resources should be activated?
What do the concepts *culture of safety*, *just culture*, and *blame-free environment* mean as they relate to the scenario?

NURSING JOURNAL: REFLECT ON YOUR PRACTICE
WHILE HONING YOUR WRITING SKILLS

Lewin's Change Theory and Role Change

Reflect on a change process in which you have been involved. What were the restraining and driving forces? Describe the role of others involved in this process and how they might have motivated you to change. As a nurse returning to school for a baccalaureate degree, describe why you feel you are in a particular stage of Lewin's *unfreezing-change-refreeze* model.

CHAPTER 6 REFERENCES

American Society for Quality. (2009). Project planning and implementing tools. http://www.asq. org/learn-about-quality/project-planning-tools/overview/pdca-cycle.html

Barnsteiner, J., Disch, J., Johnson, J., McGuinn, K., Chappell, K., & Swartwout, E. (2013). Diffusing QSEN competencies across schools of nursing: The AACN/RWJF faculty development institutes. *Journal of Professional Nursing, 29*(2), 68–74. https://doi.org/10.1016/j. profnurs.2012.12.003

Cleary, M., West, S., Arthur, D., & Kornhaber, R. (2019). Change management in health care and mental health nursing. *Issues in Mental Health Nursing, 40*(11), 966–972. https://doi.org/10.10 80/01612840.2019.1609633

Cronenwett, L., Sherwood, G., Barnsteiner J., Disch, J., Johnson, J., Mitchell, P., Sullivan, D., & Warren, J. (2007). Quality and safety education for nurses. *Nursing Outlook, 55*(3)122–131.

Doerner, M. E., & Swenty, C. F. (2019). The effect of a perioperative clinical immersion on senior nursing students' perception of readiness to practice: A quality improvement project. *AORN Journal, 109*(2), 193–200. http://dx.doi.org.ezproxy.fitchburgstate.edu:2048/10.1002/ aorn.12581

Dolansky, M. A., & Moore, S. M. (2013). Quality and safety education for nurses (QSEN): The key is systems thinking. OJIN: *The Online Journal of Issues in Nursing, 18*(3), Manuscript 1.

Emergency Care Research Institute (ECCRI). https://www.ecri.org/solutions/patient-safety-organization

Famolaro, T., Dyer, N., Burns, W., Flashner, E., Liu, H., & Sorra J. (2016). Hospital survey on patient safety culture: User comparative database report. U.S. Department of Health and Human Services, Agency for Healthcare Research and Quality (ARHQ).

Health Resources and Services Administration (HRSA) U. S. Department of Health and Human Services. (2011). *Quality improvement. Developing and implementing a QI plan.* https://www.hrsa. gov/sites/default/files/quality/toolbox/508pdfs/qualityimprovement.pdf

Institute of Medicine (IOM). (2003). *Health professions education: A bridge to quality.* National Academies Press.

Leonard, M., & Frankel, A. (2010). The path to safe and reliable healthcare. *Patient Education and Counseling, 80*(3), 288–292. https://doi.org/10.1016/j.pec.2010.07.001

Lewin, K. (1951). *Field theory in social science.* Tavistock Publications.

Maindonald, J., & Richardson, A (2004). This passionate study: A dialogue with Florence Nightingale. *Journal of Statistics Education, 12,* 1. https://.doi.org/10.1080/10691898.2004.11910718

Shirey, M. R. (2013). Lewin's theory of planned change as a strategic resource. *Journal of Nursing Administration, 43*(2), 69–72. https://doi.org/10.1097/NNA.0b013e31827f20a9

The Joint Commission (TJC). (2009) *The Joint Commission leadership standards*. Joint Commission Resources.

Wojciechowski, E., Murphy, P., Pearsall, T., & French, E. (2016). A case review: Integrating Lewin's theory with lean's system approach for change. *OJIN: The Online Journal of Issues in Nursing, 21*(2), Manuscript 4. https://doi.org/10.3912/OJIN.Vol21No02Man04

OTHER REFERENCES

Emergency Care Research Institute: https://www.ecri.org/solutions/patient-safety-organization

The Consumer Assessment of Healthcare Providers and Systems Ambulatory Care Improvement Guide: Practical Strategies for Improving Patient Experience. Content last reviewed February 2020. Agency for Healthcare Research and Quality: https://www.ahrq.gov/cahps/quality-improvement/improvement-guide/improvement-guide.html

CREDITS

Fig. 6.1: Adapted from Source: https://9mconsulting.com/newsletter/lewins-change-model/.

Fig. 6.2: Source: https://www.wevalgo.com/know-how/lean-management/lean-manufacturing.

CHAPTER 7

Utilize Informatics

CHAPTER INTRODUCTION

In this chapter, the reader is invited to reflect on how the Information Age, technological advances, and informatics have affected educational experience and nursing practice. In assuming a professional career choice of lifelong learning, nurses must adapt to continual change. Technology plays a major role in this process. A review of the literature and examples of informatics research highlights advantages and the challenges of integrating technology, as well as supports the need for continual professional development in this area among all health-care providers.

The role of the nurse informatics specialist (NIS) is highlighted in relation to supplying the tools, skills, and support of informatics implementation in the health-care setting. Telehealth nursing is integrated into the chapter as an example of acceptance of a transformative process of change affecting all stakeholders in health-care organizations.

KEY TERMS: MAKING CONNECTIONS

- Electronic Health Record (EHR)
- Health Information Portability Accountability Act (HIPAA)
- Information literacy
- IOM competency: utilize informatics
- Nurse informatics specialist (NIS)
- Telehealth/telenursing

LEARNING OBJECTIVES/OUTCOMES

At the end of this chapter, students will accomplish the following:

- Discuss the effects of informatics technology on professional practice.
- Explain the purpose of various informatics tools used in health-care delivery.
- Identify key issues related to informatics and the documentation process.
- Examine the roles of the NIS and the telehealth nurse and their effect on technology and communication for health-care providers and patients.

In God we trust. All others must bring data.

—*W. Edwards Deming, statistician, professor, author, lecturer, consultant*

If future generations are to remember us more with gratitude than sorrow,
we must achieve more than just the miracles of technology. We must also
leave them a glimpse of the world as it was created, not just as it looked when
we got through with it.

—*Lyndon B Johnson*

A NURSE'S PERSPECTIVE

I am an older "new" nurse. Many of my fellow nursing school classmates were years younger. I was an immigrant to the land of technology; they were natives. As students, we learned that although the copyright on the textbooks listed one date, the content was seven years older, and technology used at the bedside during our clinical rotations was scarcely mentioned in these texts.

In her article "Our Iceberg is Melting," Murray (2018) advocates adaptation in education: "Stop preparing tomorrow's workforce for yesterday's jobs." Nurses should be prepared for a world where the skills of data consolidation, interpretation, and dissemination are as vital as clinical skills. (RN to BS student)

NURSING INFORMATICS

In her editorial "Our Iceberg is Melting," Murray (2018) related a story about a group of penguins who must adapt to the fact that their iceberg is melting or perish. This message is a metaphor for successful adaptation to the increasingly pervasive use of informatics in society. In today's world of evolving technology, learning from a near decade-old textbook is a sign that, indeed, the iceberg is melting.

In order for informatics to be continually and effectively integrated into nursing practice, users must understand its components. Murray (2018) provided recommendations to shape the future of higher education regarding the integration of informatics. For nursing, this is recognition of the fact that the profession will continue to change and evolve as technology changes; remaining in the past is not an option. There will always be a need to modify what is already present, as new EBP is presented, as new technology comes out, and as people become more informed about their own health.

Future baccalaureate nurses, and the faculty who teach them, need to be prepared for technological development early on in the educational process. Students should be equipped with the tools they need to thrive in a world defined by technology. Students who understand this at the start of their nursing program are able to spend more time developing an understanding of the current technology, its expected advances, and its meaning for professional development and lifelong learning.

Watts (2016) recommended that an *Introduction to Nursing Informatics* course be required for all nursing programs. The curriculum should incorporate simulation experiences woven into each course associated with a clinical component, online learning exercises, discussion board communication, and exposure to open educational resources to include articles written by nurses working on the front lines of the profession. In simulation and virtual reality (VR) experiences (Medical Simulation Resources, 2018), for example, patients can be seen via the student's VR goggles. The student is able to interact with the patient to perform procedures and assessments. All of these experiences are impressive modalities that when added to such a course reinforce classroom and clinical learning, highlight student gaps in knowledge and understanding, invite reflection, and stimulate further discussion.

As technology continues to evolve, new platforms are often introduced for nurses. An example of this can be seen in the work of VISICU Inc., an organization providing health-care information technology and clinical solutions. This company offers a critical care program that allows remote monitoring of intensive care units. VISICU uses audiovisual equipment and electronic medical records to allow clinicians and providers to monitor patients remotely and to be alerted to any problems.

Nurses and other health-care providers, educators, institution and organization administrators, and students should work together to familiarize themselves with the benefits and needs of current technology. It is crucial for all stakeholders to advocate for and incorporate these technological tools and skills into their education and practice settings. Those who avoid the experience will certainly fall behind, as technological change is an inevitable reality of the profession.

KOTTER'S CHANGE MANAGEMENT THEORY

The use of Kotter's change management theory can help those tentative individuals embrace technology. Kotter's *process for leading change* was cultivated from more than 4 decades of observations of transformative leaders and organizations (Kotter, 2012). This dynamic model consists of eight stages and is organized into three phases:

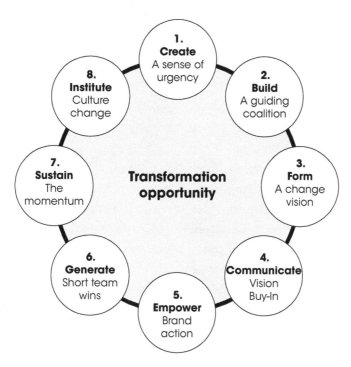

Figure 7.1 Kotter's Model

The first phase, *creating a climate for change*, includes establishing a sense of urgency, creating a guiding coalition, and developing a vision and strategy. The biggest obstacle in attempting change is complacency (Kotter, 2012). Without a sense of urgency, people will maintain the status quo and resist change. Creating urgency involves helping people see and feel firsthand why a change needs to occur. Once the vision has been created and accepted by stakeholders, the message must be disseminated compellingly, which is best achieved through frequent communication from role modeling. Group members need to hear a consistent message from everyone for both acceptance of the idea and eventual position of empowerment from which they will advocate for the change. This involves engaging in continuous dialogue with stakeholders to build commitment and trust (Neumeier, 2013).

The second phase, *engaging and enabling the organization*, incorporates the vision, empowering action, and creating a guiding coalition.Identified guiding team members must possess the knowledge, credibility, influence, and skills required to mobilize change (Kotter, 2012). Individuals work together as a team to remove obstacles and encourage everyone's participation. This may involve providing incentives for embracing change and obtaining feedback on how they can use the changes for their benefit. Changing the culture of a workplace takes time, and as time goes on, urgency drops and complacency rises (Kotter, 2012). Creating short-term goals (*wins*) maintains momentum and should be celebrated to motivate the team to create new goals. After each win, it is important to examine and analyze what worked and what needs improvement (Neumeier, 2013).

The final phase, *implementing and sustaining the change*, involves consolidating gains and producing more change and securing the new strategies into the organization's culture. The seventh and eighth stages found in this phase encompass merging strategies to effect additional change. Caution is recommended in claiming victory prematurely, as individuals may lose the sense of urgency or return to a state of complacency if changes have not been secured into the culture (Kotter, 2012). Continual focus on efforts to achieve the vision is crucial during this phase until the change becomes a permanent part of the organization's culture, which is demonstrated through its shared norms and values.

THE ROLE OF INFORMATICS TECHNOLOGY IN TRANSFORMING HEALTH CARE

The trend in the United States following the IOM report *To Err is Human: Building a Safer Health System* (IOM, 2000) was to move toward the adoption of an **EHR** as a way to transform health care and improve patient safety. The EHR provides contact with patient information and can include computerized prescriber order entry (CPOE) and electronic medication administration record functions (Neumeier, 2013). Using an EHR with CPOE improves access to more complete patient information, enhances medication safety, decreases prescribing errors, and eliminates the need for redundant data entry and the potential for error that causes (Neumeier, 2013).

Effective change management is essential to successful implementation of an EHR. Barriers to such change include high costs, lack of standardization, privacy concerns, and, most significantly, resistance to change. Implementing an EHR involves significant change, and if that change is not requested by staff, resistance may be the response. Staff acceptance of and willingness are major determinants of this innovation's success. With nurses as significant stakeholders in health care, their investment in and support of EHR implementation is an important factor in achieving success with such an undertaking.

The majority of health-care provision documentation that occurs in the EHR is completed by nurses. While time spent in the EHR reduces direct patient contact, nurse still spend more time with patients than other members of the health-care team. Since nurses work extensively with EHR, it is important to examine their experience with the technology and obtain their feedback for improving the system (Higgins et al., 2017).

Nursing leaders cite that those organizations, driven by a culture of teamwork and resiliency with change, achieve safe quality patient outcomes. In some organizations, however, nurses and their colleagues are left unsupported to master the changes that come with conquering a new EHR system. Organizations can increase user satisfaction among their nurses by soliciting their input and feedback. Regardless of a user's clinical background, an EHR can be difficult to learn, and nurses generally report room for improvement when it comes to factors related to EHR usability (Higgins et al., 2017).

Nurses have reported that the most important factors influencing the adoption of an EHR are the change management techniques used. Nurses emphasized the need to be involved in the decision-making process from the beginning as part of project teams and usability testing. When they are not included in shared decision making, the EHR cannot adequately support their work. Neglecting to manage the human side of technology implementation presents serious challenges, which can ultimately lead to failure of the EHR to be adopted (Higgins et al., 2017).

Developing a strategy for successful EHR implementation and evaluation should incorporate all participants. The organization's vision statement originally created during the development of the EHR should be reevaluated to ensure that it is still current, realistic, and service oriented. At the same time, any changes to the vision should be shared with all group members. In this way, the goal is not simply about EHR acceptance related to efficiency and cost containment but also includes the motivation and collective buy-in of all stakeholders (Campbell, 2008).

THE NURSE INFORMATICS SPECIALIST

With her meticulous record keeping during the Crimean War, Florence Nightingale is often referred to as the first informatics nurse. She sought to improve conditions for soldiers on the battlefield using patient data to guide her work. Because of her detailed documentation and presentation of this information, Nightingale significantly improved the nursing care provided to British soldiers in Crimea. Nightingale demonstrated that with well-documented information, patient care can be improved (Kirchner, 2014).

The ANA defines informatics nursing as the integration of nursing with analytical sciences to identify, define, manage, and communicate data, information, knowledge, and wisdom in nursing practice (ANA, 2014). Nursing informatics encompasses a diverse array of nursing strengths and interests. It affects virtually every aspect of health care where technology integrates with clinical practice, regardless of the setting. Nurses who pursue informatics as a career expand their reach beyond direct patient care, but they still experience the rewards of helping people and advocating for their profession

The **nurse informatics specialist (NIS)** is an RN with extensive clinical experience who possesses additional knowledge and skills related to technology and information systems. From the Healthcare Information and Management Systems Society (HIMSS) *2014 Nursing Informatics* survey (HIMSS, 2017), 58% of NIS respondents stated that their experience with informatics education came from on-the-job training. However, according the HIMSS survey, 60% of the respondents possessed a postgraduate degree in informatics or other field or specialty. The survey also noted that 19% of the respondents had a certificate in nursing informatics from a postgraduate education program or by successfully passing the AACN certification test (Kirchner, 2014).

The unique skill set that the NIS possesses is invaluable for dealing with an institution's technology. Through the application of nursing clinical knowledge and the understanding of computer and information sciences, the NIS brings a nursing perspective to the integration of clinical applications into nursing workflow and patient care. Because of the insights of nurse informaticists into clinical needs and understanding of the EHR system, they can communicate to the technical staff about the ongoing needs of nurses who are using the EHR. The NIS is an advocate and voice for nurses in matters involving the EHR and other applications of technology to nursing care (Kirchner, 2014).

Every 3 years, the HIMSS conducts a nursing informatics workforce survey to gain insight into the specialty. Nelson and Parker (2019) published a summary of data gathered from the 2011, 2014, and 2017 surveys, which highlighted clinical experience, training and education, and roles and responsibilities:

> Clinical experience is integral for success in informatics nursing; 82% of respondents reported working in a clinical setting for more than five years before switching to informatics. The most commonly reported care settings were medical-surgical, critical care, emergency, pediatrics, and administration. Of the informatics nurses who responded, 80% report that they are "highly satisfied" with their career choice. (Nelson & Parker, 2019)

Regarding training and education, Nelson and Parker (2019) reported a shift from on-the-job training to receiving master's and doctoral degrees and postgraduate certificates. The two specialized roles are the informatics RN (with experience working in health information technology) and informatics nurse specialist (with health IT experience and a master's or doctorate degree). Board certification through the American Nurses Credentialing Center, professional certification through HIMSS, and project management certifications are common and beneficial qualifications for one's nursing career goals.

In the area of roles and responsibilities, a nursing informatics career creates a pathway for advancing nursing science. With health-care technology innovation, design and implementation responsibilities grow (Nelson & Parker, 2019). In their search for value, efficiency, and seamless experience for health-care providers, many health-care organizations are already replacing their former EHRs with systems better suited to their needs. Informatics nurses entering such a system use their skills to help create and implement systems that support the clinician's voice in their designs. At this point, the NIS supports a transformative process in the educator role.

Nurses desire an EHR that is intuitive, user-friendly, and easy to troubleshoot. With background and knowledge, the NIS can effect change by serving as a bridge between technology and nurses' clinical needs. It should be noted that the informatics nurse must be cognizant of the need to function as a member of the team, in collaboration with other staff members (Kirchner, 2014).

As a link between technology and patient care, the NIS is employed in hospitals, universities, consulting firms, or other health-care organizations. Within these institutions, the NIS is visible in all areas of patient care, from acute inpatient care and ambulatory home health areas to telehealth settings. Among diverse health-care organizations and settings, administrators recognize the full potential of the nurse informaticist to improve the quality of patient care and reduce costs (Kirchner, 2014).

Francis (2017) reported that nursing informatics is fundamentally based on the principle of nursing as a caring science. Caring is central in the practice of technology. When NISs advocate caring as a core nursing value supported by technology, they convey an important message to patients and their fellow health-care providers.

The role of the NIS continues to develop to enhance the connection between health-care providers and patients (Nagle et al., 2017). Initially, the role of the NIS focused on supporting the purchase of EHR systems, along with their implementation and maintenance in health-care organizations. With the growth of telehealth in ambulatory settings, it is an expectation for the NIS to offer those same skills in a different environment. Nagle et al. (2017) stressed that nursing input and informatics expertise and support are crucial to ensuring appropriate, quality, and safe use of these tools in the telehealth domain. As patients become more active participants in their care via the telehealth model to communicate with providers, they need the support and expertise of the NIS to steer them in the right direction.

TELEHEALTH AND TELENURSING

Current technology enables nurses to reach out to patients in isolated settings, monitor their conditions, and interact with them using computers, audiovisual equipment, and telephones. **Telehealth** is the use of electronic information and telecommunications technology to support remote clinical health care, patient and professional health-related education, public health, and health administration. With the success of telehealth in specialty health-care services, the use of this technology to transmit health information and provide care remotely has now found its way to mainstream health service delivery (Bashir & Bastola, 2018).

Telehealth nursing significantly affects patient care, particularly in rural or underserved areas with shortages of nurses, health-care services, and resources. For home health agencies serving the homebound and vulnerable patient populations, telehealth capability is invaluable. This model can significantly alleviate gaps in health-care services, ultimately reducing stress for this patient population.

The current *AAACN Scope and Standards of Practice for Professional Telehealth Nursing* (2018) offers guiding principles for telenursing practice to recognize patient needs and identify those resources available to meet desired outcomes. According to West and Artinian (2019), the role of the telenurse in supporting patients has grown concurrently with the expansion of technology in the nursing profession. However, the authors report that many patients are initially hesitant to use the telehealth model and recommend the proactive support of telenurses to encourage the use of telehealth for their care needs.

Telehealth nursing does not necessarily require certification. Telehealth nurses must possess a RN license that complies with federal as well as state regulations. All telehealth nurses must practice within the ANA standards for safety and quality as well as competency. Specific telehealth standards are available at the American Academy of Ambulatory Care Nurses and the ANA (2014; AAACN, 2018). Nurses who offer telehealth services must maintain patient confidentiality and observe HIPAA requirements that apply to this branch of nursing practice (Borten, 2019).

It is important to evaluate the quality of service from those health professionals involved in telehealth, as well as the process itself, when managing nursing care services provided through this technology. A pilot study conducted by researchers Bashir and Bastola (2018) sought to examine whether telehealth technology affected a perceived level of internal service quality delivered by nurses within a telehealth organization. Although previous studies assessed the cost-effectiveness and patient acceptance of this method of service delivery, the perspective of nurses as service providers had not been investigated.

The aim of the study by Bashir and Bastola (2018) was to investigate telehealth nursing service quality (TNSQ) from the nurses' perspective. To address this research goal, the authors developed and empirically tested the notion of TNSQ. Data were collected from nurses working in a home care agency based on interview questions related to TNSQ. Follow-up interviews were conducted to validate questions on the revised instrument.

The findings of this study (Bashir & Bastola, 2018) were positive, based on mean differences between expectations and perceptions of TNSQ. The responses to the interview questions and data gathered from the survey showed overall satisfaction with TNSQ. The study highlighted how the telehealth process provides daily monitoring of patient health, leading to the benefits of immediate feedback for patients, family, and caregivers, as well as convenience of scheduling.

Integration of inpatient EHRs in health-care organizations across the United States is commonplace today. Although EHR and telehealth technology has been readily accepted and integrated into rural areas and determined useful for chronic disease monitoring, telehealth adoption has been slow in urban primary care settings. The aim of a study by West and Artinian (2019) was to elicit the perceptions of adult patients in an urban setting when telehealth encounters were available. A qualitative study design was employed to collect data through interviews from 21 patients in a primary care practice. Interview questions included (a) How do patients select any type of appointment? (b) How do patients perceive and use telehealth options? (c) How and when might telehealth be useful in the future? (West & Artinian, 2019).

A theory of *weighing options* emerged. In weighing their options for choosing a telehealth encounter and seeking care, patients balance those *hassle factors*, such as urgency, timing, scheduling, transpersonal relationships, distance, and convenience. Of the considerations made when weighing options, the transpersonal relationship was primary in patients' decisions. Implications from this study for nurses and other health-care providers include enabling awareness of and support for patients when onboarding and employing telehealth encounters. Research data from patients' perspectives can promote strategies for telenurses, NIS, and other health-care providers to help patients make the decision to choose telehealth encounters (West & Artinian, 2019). To realize the potential of telehealth, Fathi et al. (2017) cite the need for new practice models where ambulatory care and informatics nurses train and work in advanced roles to lead telehealth integration into practices.

To determine staff competencies in telehealth, van Houwelingen et al. (2016) organized nurses, nursing faculty, clients, and technicians in a Delphi study. The team identified six core competencies with *nursing telehealth entrustable professional activities* and knowledge, attitudes, and skills required across those activities. Examples of such activities include supporting and educating patients in the use of technology to strengthen their social networks. The authors highlight those telehealth competencies with corresponding skills. Increased engagement by primary care patients could be realized by incorporating these skills into practice by the telenurse or NIS (van Houwelingen et al., 2016).

TELEHEALTH COMPETENCIES WITH CORRESPONDING SKILLS

Knowledge

- Knowledge of the (clinical) limitations of telehealth
- Knowledge about what to do if the technology does not work

Attitudes

- Conveys empathy through videoconferencing by facial expression and verbal communication
- Promotes privacy and confidentiality in videoconferencing
- Enhances the confidence of the patient in the deployed technology

Technological skills

- Trains the patient to use the equipment
- Checks equipment for functionality

Communication skills

- Communicates clearly in videoconferencing and knows what to do to enhance contact (e.g., use of voice, light, background)
- Puts patients at ease when they feel insecure about using technology

Implementation skills

- Assesses whether telehealth is convenient for the patient by the use of established criteria (for example, cognitive ability, technological skills)

NURSING AND HIPAA

Nurses deal with private information daily, regardless of the health-care setting. With a focus on patient health and exposure to constant contact with patient data, nurses risk becoming desensitized to the importance of protecting the digital and physical paper trail. The reality is that all patient information is confidential and federally protected.

In 1996, HIPAA was introduced as a federal law to uphold a national set of standards for the confidential and secure electronic exchange of personal health information by the healthcare industry. The "Privacy and Security Rules" section is an important element of HIPAA (Borten, 2019). This work delineates how nurses and other providers should collect, use, and handle protected health information (PHI).

Nurses are introduced to HIPAA as students, early on in their nursing curriculum. It is crucial to possess a full understanding of patient privacy laws early on in classroom and clinical education. With the increased use of electronic devices, sensitive data are at risk of being compromised. All health-care providers must be vigilant in following HIPAA guidelines to ensure that patients' private records are protected from any unauthorized distribution (Cataletto, 2011).

There are a number of actions nurses can take to improve the security and privacy of patient information in the workplace. The biggest adjustment, spanning all tasks, facilities, and responsibilities, involves situational awareness (Borten, 2019). For nurses, discussing patient care is essential in most cases; however, the potential exists for an individual's health information to be disclosed unintentionally. Conversation is a normal part of the workplace, but nurses should avoid sharing patient information unless approved under HIPAA guidelines. Nurses, too, need to ensure that their mobile devices are password protected. Also, they should avoid posting comments or photographs related to the workplace. In particular, nurses should be aware of the security policies and procedures involved in the proper handling of information (Cataletto, 2011).

Per the privacy rule, specific disclosures of PHI may occur when policies and procedures are in place to protect an individual's privacy, such as lowering one's voice when sharing patient information with staff members and patients' families, especially in a public setting. It may also include privacy filters installed on computer screens to safeguard patient information from being viewed by bystanders. In handling hard copies of records, papers and files must not be visible at the nurse's station but secured in a locked drawer or file cabinet. Record rooms also should be kept locked when unattended, with access limited to authorized personnel only. Physical documents no longer needed should be shredded (Borten, 2019).

Digitalized medical records create readily available patient information for health-care providers. However, keeping this information secure can prove to be challenging. From nursing station monitors, to laptops on a mobile cart (*computers on wheels*), to tablets in examination rooms, PHI is readily accessible on countless computer screens.

Nurses play a crucial role in protecting patients and their personal health information. But the effort is not solely on these caregivers. All health-care providers must commit to following security and privacy policies to help create the first line of defense in protecting confidential patient information.

CHAPTER SUMMARY

In this chapter, readers were introduced to the latest trends in health-care related to the IOM competency of using informatics. The rapid and ever-changing technological advances in health care and their effect on nurses' clinical practice, autonomy, responsibility, and professionalism was presented through the presentation of current literature. Content in this chapter reinforced the importance of computer literacy, lifelong learning, and an EBP philosophy as key professional nursing skills. A review of Kotter's change management theory reinforces both advantages and challenges of adaptation to change as it relates to informatics technology in nursing and health care. An overview of the specialized roles of the telenurse and the NIS provided additional evidence of the opportunities available for career advancement, professional development, and job satisfaction.

FOOD FOR THOUGHT: CRITICAL THINKING QUESTIONS

1. What types of technology are now used in hospitals to avoid potential medication errors?
2. Describe benefits and limitations of technology (barcodes, automatic alarms, EHR, telemedicine)
3. Discuss the implications of "work arounds" in patient care. What types of policies should exist for those taking shortcuts in medication administration?

SCENARIO: APPLYING WHAT YOU HAVE LEARNED

Informatics and Documentation

In the intensive care unit at their hospital, nurses use the "VISICU" electronic documentation system. The assessment portion evaluates each client using a system approach similar to nursing theorist Callista Roy's adaptation model and the first level of assessment: physiologic-physical mode, where nurses assess and note items such as oxygenation, safety, and level of neurological functioning. Care plans are updated each shift and include areas such as the client's disposition, safety, and nutritional needs. A "free-text" section allows for documentation of client-specific issues. The method of approach to this section uses Roy's model: nursing diagnoses, patient-specific intervention, patient-specific goals, and means of evaluation are listed.

Recently widowed 70-year-old client Martin Allen arrives at his physician's office with shortness of breath related to a medical diagnosis of congestive heart failure. He has stopped taking his prescribed Lasix medication, stating it makes him urinate frequently. He admits to noncompliance with his diet, eating most of his meals at the local fast-food restaurant.

1. What would you document in his electronic record?
2. What would you document in the "free-text" section?

3. What nursing diagnosis/diagnoses correlate to Mr. Allen's current status?
4. What goals does the nurse discuss with Mr. Allen and with the health-care team?
5. What specific interventions will meet these goals?
6. How would the nurse evaluate if the goals were met?
7. According to Roy's theory, how is the client coping?
8. How does coping affect his present state?

NURSING JOURNAL: REFLECT ON YOUR PRACTICE WHILE HONING YOUR WRITING SKILLS

Information Literacy

Information literacy is the ability to recognize when information is needed and possessing the capacity to locate, evaluate, and use the needed information effectively (Schloman, 2001). The information literate individual is an information consumer who believes in lifelong learning. We are surrounded by communication and information technologies that allow access to extensive reservoirs of information that are useful only if we know how to capitalize on them. Knowing how to seek, evaluate, and apply information is critical to ensure ongoing professional competence. With this in mind, construct a narrative that integrates your responses to the following questions:

- How does information literacy relate to nursing?
- What are the components of information literacy?
- Why is information literacy an essential skill for the RN in their daily practice?
- Why is digital literacy important for nurses?
- Why is health-care literacy important for everyone?

CHAPTER 7 REFERENCES

American Academy of Ambulatory Care Nursing (AAACN). (2018). *Scope and standards of practice for professional telehealth nursing* (6th ed.).

American Nurses Association (ANA). (2014). Nursing informatics: Scope and standards of practice (2nd ed.).

Bashir, A., & Bastola, D. R. (2018). Perspectives of nurses toward telehealth efficacy and quality of health care: A pilot study. *JMIR Medical Informatics, 6*(2), e35. https://doi.org/10.2196/medinform.9080

Borten, K. (2016). The role of Nurses in HIPAA compliance, healthcare security. *HIPAA and Compliance News,* 1–3.

Campbell, R. J. (2008). Change management in health care. *Health Care Manager, 27*(1), 23–39.

Cataletto, M. (2011). Highlights of HIPAA for nurses. *Nursing Made Incredibly Easy, 9* (3), 6–8. https://doi.org/10.1097/01.NME.0000396003.87676.52

Fathi, J. T., Modin, H. E., & Scott, J. D. (2019). Nurses advancing telehealth services in the era of healthcare reform. *OJIN: The Online Journal of Issues in Nursing, 22*(2). https://doi.org/10.3912/OJIN.Vol22No02Man0

Francis, I. (2017). Nursing informatics and the metaparadigms of nursing. *Online Journal of Nursing Informatics, 21*(1), 8–1.

Healthcare Information and Management Systems Society (HIMSS). (2017). Nursing informatics workforce survey. himss.org/sites/himssorg/files/2017nursing-informatics-workforce-full-report.pdf

Higgins, L., Shovel, J., Bilderback, A., Lorenz, H; Martin, S., Rogers, D., & Minnier, T. (2017). Hospital nurses' work activity in a technology-rich environment: A triangulated quality improvement assessment. *Journal of Nursing Care Quality, 32*(3), 208–217. https://doi.org/10.1097/NCQ.0000000000000237.

Institute of Medicine (IOM). (2000). *To err is human: Building a safer health system.* National Academies Press. https://doi.org/10.17226/9728.

Kirchner, R. (2014). Introducing nursing informatics. *Nursing 2014, 44*(9), 22–23. https://doi.org/10.1097/01.NURSE.0000453006.79653.33

Kotter, J. P. (2012). *Leading change.* Harvard Business Review Press.

Medical Simulation Resources. (2018). Simulation for health provides VR training for healthcare. *Nursing Informatics Today, 31*(1), 10–16. https://www.youtube.com/watch?v=3y56gr_27ro&feature=emb_rel_end

Murray, T. A. (2018). Nursing education: Our iceberg is melting.*Journal of Nursing Education,57,* 575–576.

Nagle, L., Sermeus, W., & Junger, A. (2017). Evolving role of the nursing informatics specialist. *Studies in Health Technology and Informatics, 232,* 212–221.

Nelson, T., & Parker, C. (2019). Nursing informatics: The EHR and beyond. *American Nurse Today, (14)*3, 36–38.

Neumeier, M. (2013). Using Kotter's change management theory and innovation diffusion theory implementing an electronic medical record (EMR). *Canadian Journal of Nursing Informatics, 8* (1 & 2).

Schloman, B. (2001). Information resources: Information literacy: The benefits of partnership. *Online Journal of Issues in Nursing.* www.nursingworld.org/MainMenuCategories/ANAMarketplace/ANAPeriodicals/OJIN/Columns/InformationResources/InformationLiteracy.aspx

van Houwelingen, C., Moerman, A., Ettema, R., Kort, H., & Ten, C. (2016). Competencies required for nursing telehealth activities: A Delphi-study. *Nurse Education Today, 39,* 50–62. https://doi.org/10.1016/j.nedt.2015.12.025

Watts, C. S. (2016). Preparing nursing graduates for the future: Adding informatics education to entry level Programs. *Nursing Informatics Today, 31*(1), 10–16.

West, K., & Artinian, B. (2019). Weighing options: Perceptions of adult patients accessing tele-health in primary care. *OJNI: The Online Journal of Nursing Informatics, 23*(3). http://www.himss.org/ojni

CREDIT